7-DAY KETO DIET MEAL PLAN

Fresh and healthy Keto instant pot recipes cookbook

HAILEY.T

ISBN: 9781799030225

TEXT COPYRIGHT © [HAILEY.T]

Legal & Disclaimer

The information contained in this book and its contents is not designed to replace or take the place of any form of medical or professional advice; and is not meant to replace the need for independent medical, financial, legal or other professional advice or services, as may be required. The content and information in this book has been provided for educational purposes only.

The content and information contained in this book has been compiled from sources deemed reliable, and it is accurate to the best of the Author's knowledge, information and belief. However, the Author cannot guarantee its accuracy and validity and cannot be held liable for any errors and/or omissions. Further, changes are periodically made to this book as and when needed. Where appropriate and/or necessary, you must consult a professional (including but not limited to your doctor, attorney, financial advisor or such other professional advisor) before using any of the suggested remedies, techniques, or information in this book.

Upon using the contents and information contained in this book, you agree to hold harmless the Author from and against any damages, costs, and expenses, including any legal fees potentially resulting from the application of any of the information provided by this book. This disclaimer applies to any loss, damages or injury caused by the use and application, whether directly or indirectly, of any advice or information presented, whether for breach of contract, tort, negligence, personal injury, criminal intent, or under any other cause of action.

You agree to accept all risks of using the information presented inside this book.

You agree that by continuing to read this book, where appropriate and/or necessary, you shall consult a professional (including but not limited to your doctor, attorney, or financial advisor or such other advisor as needed) before using any of the suggested remedies, techniques, or information in this book.

Table of Contents

Introduction

Healthy living is not just a dream for our modern generation, but it has become a necessary factor to stay in tune with our modern, fast-paced lifestyle. Obesity, weight gain, heart diseases, diabetes, and many other critical health disorders are on the serious high rise. The ketogenic diet is aimed to take control of your food and consume nutritionally balanced meals to counter such essential diseases of health.

Ketogenic Diet, also popularly referred as a keto diet, is a unique form of eating that focuses on reducing the consumption of bad carbohydrates. It is focused on maximizing the consumption of healthy fats and protein to transform our overall health. The ketogenic diet promotes healthy weight loss by triggering the process of ketosis; ketosis aims to replace healthy fats instead of stored carbohydrates as a primary source of energy. Our body is prompted to utilize healthy fats for energy requirements, and it helps to improve our health in many ways including promoting natural weight loss.

Instant Pot cooking has become the most popular and effective way of preparing everyday recipes. Millions of people are relying on Instant Pot to make healthy and delicious meals in a matter of minutes.

Instant Pot is the perfect cooking partner to start your ketogenic diet. It saves you from all the troubles of cooking by converting complex cooking tasks into easy to follow steps. It makes it easier for you to stay focused on ketogenic diet and rip its health benefits. Instant Pot prepared nutrient rich ketogenic meals in real quick time for your whole family. It preserves nutrition and gives you nutritionally balanced meals every day.

This dedicated book on Instant Pot keto diet unveils a hand-picked collection of ketogenic diet recipes for beginners. The recipes are easy to prepare to suit beginners with easy to follow recipe instructions. Moreover, the recipes are quick to cook using an Instant Pot.

Get ready to learn to prepare a variety of ketogenic recipes at home using an Instant Pot and lead a truly healthy lifestyle. Let's get started.

A ketogenic diet will drastically reduce your daily carb intake and replace it with healthy fat. The reduction of carb helps the body to assume a state known as ketosis.

In this condition, the body becomes extremely efficient and burns fat for energy. It also helps to transform fat into ketones in the liver, which results in supplying energy to the brain.

With a ketogenic diet, one can experience huge reductions in insulin levels and blood sugar. The increased number of ketones includes a number of health benefits.

A number of versions of the ketogenic diet are noted:

•   Standard ketogenic diet or SKD is a moderate-protein, low-carb, and high-fat diet, which contains 20% protein, 75% carbs, and 5% fat.

•   Targeted ketogenic diet or TKD includes carbs around workouts.

•   Cyclical ketogenic diet or CKD allows you to have higher carb refeeds like 5 intense ketogenic days followed by 2 high-carb days.

•   The high-protein ketogenic diet is almost like a standard ketogenic diet with the only exception of including more protein. The ratio stands at 60% fat, 5% carb, and 35% protein.

Cyclical and targeted ketogenic diets are more advanced and usually are given to athletes and bodybuilders.

A ketogenic diet is one of the effective ways to lose weight and decrease factors for disease such as high pressure and high blood sugar. It has been found out that people in a ketogenic diet have lost 2.2 times more weight than those in a calorie-restricted low-fat diet.

Apart from regular diseases, the ketogenic diet has also proved to be beneficial for several types of cancer and slow the growth of the tumor. It has also shown remarkable progress in people who have Alzheimer's disease; the diet has slowed the development of the disease.

Women suffering from PCOS or polycystic ovary syndrome have seen a remarkable decrease in their insulin levels. Once the insulin levels are decreased, one can see a remarkable improvement in the outbreak of acne.

Chapter 1: Is the Keto Diet Right for You?

Although I recommend the ketogenic diet, the results may vary from person to person. While following this or any other diet, you need to know what is suitable for you. You will need to ask yourself some questions before you decide to get started.

Firstly, this diet is more beneficial for people who are solely looking to lose excess fat from their body at first. If you are on another diet or have previously tried other diets, consider how you feel while on it. Do you keep feeling hungry and crave more food? This is quite probable if you eat carb-loaded meals. You might eat a huge dinner but within an hour or so you will crave a snack while on such diets. The keto diet will benefit you in this case because it helps to control hunger pangs and will regulate your blood sugar and insulin levels.

Due to a habitual diet, some people don't feel satisfied with their meals unless they include heavy carbs. They always need some bread or rice or other carbs on their plate. People such as these compulsively eat carbs in order to achieve that bloated feeling that carbs provide; however, it is a very unhealthy way to eat. Loading up on fats instead of carbs will give you the same satisfaction or better but in a healthier way. You will also stay full for longer because fats take longer to burn off than carbs.

The keto diet works for both lazy and disciplined people. Some people like to work on instinct when considering the food they eat while others prefer specific markers set for what their meals should consist of. This adjustable aspect of the keto diet makes it suitable for all types of people.

A ketogenic diet will slowly help you get rid of bad food habits. The processed food diet most people follow cause untimely cravings. There are people who feel quite restless if they don't have certain snacks or sweets every single day. This unhealthy food addiction can be very damning for the body and mostly consists of empty calories. Once you start reducing the carbohydrates in your diet and eating more fats, you will slowly get your body accustomed to breaking off the carb addiction. This will help you lose fat and maintain a healthy weight long-term.

It is easy to stick to a keto diet because the main parts of the meal such as meat, fish, and vegetables are not prohibited. The diet is only difficult for those who are too dependent on bread or such starchy foods in their meals. People who are overweight usually have a problem staying motivated to continue a diet. This is why strict diets often result in failure, but the keto diet can be a bit simpler for you compared to these diets. Keep track of your results in the first couple of weeks where you will first lose water weight. Slowly you will see the fat shedding from all parts of your body. Progress will be the best motivation for you to stay on the diet long-term.

The ketogenic diet is especially recommended for those suffering from type 2 diabetes. This disease can cause a lot of health issues but is reversible if you follow the right diet. The keto diet helps to eliminate all sugar and carbs from your diet so your blood glucose levels are regulated. Within the first few months of following the keto diet itself, you will see improvement in your condition. It is very important to stay away from sugar in this condition and the keto diet already tells you how it affects you negatively.

The keto diet will work for you only if you stay dedicated for long enough. Unlike other fad diets, it does not promise you instant gratifying results. The goal is more long-term and so you need to stay patient and watch as it works on your body.

Precautions

Just like any other diet, consult a doctor before you follow the ketogenic diet. Your body is different from others and has its own special needs. There are certain conditions in which a particular diet might not be suitable for you. This is why a health screen is necessary to determine if you should follow the ketogenic diet or not.

The ketogenic diet is not recommended for people with kidney, liver or pancreatic diseases. There are other conditions like muscular dystrophy as well, which make it unsuitable for those people. If you have type 1 diabetes, the keto diet is completely unsuitable for you. In the case of diabetes type 2, it works for some and is not appropriate for others. You should consult your doctor to determine this. If you have gestational diabetes as well, keto is not the diet for you.

Women who are pregnant or nursing are also recommended to stay away from such diets. Such conditions require very healthy and nutritious diets and need to be accommodating to the child as well. People who suffer from eating disorders also need to be more careful about any diet they try. It is more important to focus on teaching healthy eating habits first. Going on any strict diet might not be helpful.

As you can see, there are certain conditions that make a particular diet unsuitable for your body. The goal is to help your body stay healthy and reach an appropriate weight using the right diet for you. As long as you don't suffer from the above-mentioned conditions, the keto diet will definitely be a good choice for you.

Chapter 2: Ketogenic Diet: Food List

<u>Foods to Eat</u>

Following are the foods that are emphasized on a keto diet.

- Healthy, fatty fish such as tuna, salmon, etc.

- Healthy oils such as avocado oil, coconut oil, olive oil, etc.

- All types of full-fat cheese and full-fat cream cheese, sour cream, crème Fraiche.

- Unsweetened almond/coconut milk, or other nut milk

- Eggs

- Butter, total fat

- Avocados

- Walnuts, almonds, cashews, and other nuts

- Chia seed and flax seed

- Olives

- Bacon

- Unsweetened beverages

- Heavy cream

- Healthy low carb, non-starchy veggies such as leek, fennel, spinach, kale, broccoli, tomatoes, other greens, etc.

- All types of berries but in small quantities

- Herbs and most spices

Foods to Avoid

- All types of sweetened beverages, fruit juices, and other sweetened drinks.

- All types of starchy vegetables including white potatoes, sweet potatoes, etc.

- Commercial fried foods, snacks, and bakery products including sugar-based desserts.

- Wheat pasta, bread, rice, cereals, and other high carb wheat products.

- All types of commercial processed food items.

- Legumes and beans

- Fruits can be consumed but a small quantity

- Alcohol and unhealthy cooking oils

Chapter 3: Benefits and Risks of the Keto Diet

In this chapter, let's take a look at the several benefits of this diet. Believe me, weight loss is not the only benefit of this diet. You will see shortly how this singular diet is capable of addressing several risk factors all at once. This chapter will only leave you with more reassurance that you have done the right thing by choosing this diet.

Recent research has found that the Keto Diet may be associated with some improvements in some cardiovascular risk factors, such as obesity, type 2 diabetes and HDL cholesterol levels although long-term research is not currently available.

Regulates Your Appetite

Most often the reason why I have ended up giving up on a diet plan is because I would feel so tired but mostly hungry. Most diets that I have attempted to follow in the past were so restrictive that I hardly had the satisfaction of eating enough and feeling full.

Keto diet make you feel famished beyond the first few days when your body is still getting used to fat as the source of its energy. When your body starts burning the fat stored, you will feel energized and the high fat content makes you feel full.

It doesn't feel like you are actually dieting because you still get to eat most of the things that you love except maybe your carbs. Unlike carbs, fat doesn't get digested quickly so you feel full longer.

Therefore, you won't feel hungry so often. When you consume more carbs, especially high glycemic carbs, your body burns them off quickly and you end up feeling hungry soon enough. By implementing this diet, you are actually taking care of these random hunger pains and regulating your appetite with fat and high-fiber, low glycemic vegetables.

Regulating your appetite also plays an important role in helping you lose weight. When you don't feel hungry often you will end up eating less than before and reducing the number of calories you consume. Therefore, you only have to worry about an increased number of calories to burn.

Helps in Managing Your Blood Sugar Levels

We have already seen how the intake of carbs is responsible for the release of glucose into your bloodstream. This is the reason why we immediately experience a surge in our energy levels when we consume carbs.

As you know, the hormone called ***insulin*** is responsible for regulating our blood sugar levels. However, insulin doesn't function as it is supposed to for certain people. It doesn't regulate the blood sugar levels which ultimately results in ***Type 2 diabetes***.

This phenomenon of insulin not functioning properly over a long period of time **is known as "insulin resistance"**. Recent research has shown that Insulin resistance is a primary cause for cardiovascular disease risk.

Therefore, if you are insulin resistant, the Keto Diet can help you alleviate the risk of type 2 diabetes. This is because the amount of sugar released into your bloodstream is reduced as a result of reduced intake of carbs. Even if your insulin doesn't function the way it is intended to, your blood sugar levels won't increase and you probably don't have to worry about Type-2 diabetes.

The Keto Diet is suitable even if you are suffering from Type 2 diabetes. It can actually help you manage your diabetes with minimal medication thanks to the reduced production of sugar/glucose.

Helps in Regulating Your Blood Pressure Levels

Hypertension has become a common household problem these days. This is responsible for increasing your risk factors for various disorders related to the kidneys, cardiac disorders, etc. Therefore, you simply cannot afford to turn a blind eye to hypertension.

One of the common suggestions prescribed by physicians, as part of treating hypertension, is to reduce your intake of salt. This is because salt is capable of increasing your blood pressure levels.

Well, not all of us can take this suggestion with a pinch of salt, can we? Your meals won't taste the same without adding salt to them.

Here is the good news – you don't have to cut back on your salt intake as long as it is not excessive if you are following this diet.

The Keto Diet helps in managing your blood pressure levels even without reducing your intake of salt. Let's look at how this diet is capable of doing this:

- *When you are consuming foods which are rich in carbs, your blood sugar levels will automatically increase.* When there is a surge in your blood sugar levels and if you are insulin resistant, it ends up constricting your blood vessels. The constriction in the blood vessels has an impact on your blood pressure levels and causes it to increase.

- *By reducing your carb intake, you are essentially managing your blood sugar levels.* When your blood sugar is under control, you don't have to worry about constricted blood vessels or hypertension unless you have a specific underlying condition that is causing the hypertension.

- *An important reason behind hypertension is insulin resistance.* We just saw how the Keto Diet plays an important role in managing your insulin resistance by making you reduce your intake of carbs.

- You will see in a bit how the Keto Diet helps to reduce the amount of visceral fat stored in our bodies. *The reduction in the amount of visceral fat helps in managing your insulin resistance.* This also helps to lower your risk when it comes to several cardiac disorders. With insulin resistance managed, you are reducing one more risk factor for hypertension.

- You already know that the Keto Diet encourages the body to burn the fat stored in your body. *As part of burning the fat, the sodium and potassium content in your kidneys get flushed out.*

- This results in an electrolyte imbalance, which can be addressed by the increased intake of salt and bone broth, beef broth and chicken broth. *As you can see, you are actually managing your hypertension with this diet, without reducing your intake of salt.*

Helps to Get Rid of Visceral Fat

When your body digests the foods that you consume, the fat present gets deposited in different parts of your body but you have no control over where it goes. Depending on the places where your fat gets deposited, the associated risk factors will vary. The fat that we consume gets stored under our skin **(subcutaneous fat)** or gets deposited in the abdominal cavity **(visceral fat).**

It is also capable of affecting the manner in which the different organs in your body function due to the crowding of your organs due to the visceral fat.

When there is an increase in the amount of visceral fat deposited in your body, it causes inflammation of organs. Insulin resistance and also impairs your body's metabolism. **When the metabolism of your body is impacted, your efforts to lose weight will also be impacted.** In fact, it will take you longer than usual to lose weight.

Therefore you have to make sure that your visceral fat deposits are under control.

The Keto Diet is capable of reducing the visceral fat stored in our bodies. This stubborn fat is digested by the body to derive energy. By getting rid of excess visceral fat, you are actually reducing your risk factors for various health disorders. Your efforts to lose weight will also not be compromised by the presence of visceral fat.

Risks and Side Effects to Consider – The "Keto Flu" Symptoms During Transition

While there are numerous benefits to adopting the Keto Diet (really the Keto Lifestyle), I would be remiss if I didn't make you aware of some of the risks. As with any lifestyle and diet change, you need to be fully informed to make the best decision for yourself. If you don't feel well or think that something isn't right, stop your Keto Diet immediately and please see your medical doctor right away. Don't ever take any chances.

A common occurrence when you start on the Keto Diet are a variety of symptoms often referred to as the ***"Keto Flu"***. Temporary symptoms occur as your body adapts from a high carbohydrate diet to a low carbohydrate diet as your body's glucose is depleting and your body starts to produce and use fat as energy.

Some of the common, ***temporary health changes and side effects*** that may occur when you adopt the Keto Diet include the following although this list is not meant to be comprehensive and may be different by each person:

- Body Aches and Muscle Cramps
- Headaches and Fatigue
- Dizziness and Drowsiness
- **Nausea**

- Diarrhea

To minimize and to better manage the ***"Keto Flu" symptoms***, here are a few key recommendations:

- Drink plenty of water and stay hydrated. Add some salt to your daily intake to replenish the salt that is being flushed out your system on the Keto Diet. You might also consider drinking bone, beef or chicken broth instead of adding salt.
- Consume foods high in magnesium and potassium such as dairy, leafy green vegetables, broccoli, avocados, nuts as well as various meat proteins. Include homemade bone broth. This is to replenish key nutrients and electrolytes.
- Ensure you are getting enough fats into your diet and not just focused on reducing carbohydrates. This is a common situation for those who are new to the Keto Diet.
- Get adequate rest and sleep. Don't do any strenuous exercise during the first couple of weeks but do get out and get some fresh air with daily walks.

The symptoms will typically resolve themselves between two to three weeks. If these symptoms are too much for you initially, slow down your transition to the Keto Diet and adjust to what your body is telling you.

Risks and Side Effects to Consider – Bad Breath (Ketosis Breath) As you may be aware of, a common complaint of the Keto Diet is having bad breath as the result of your body utilizing fat instead of glucose from carbohydrates for energy by the creation of ketones. Without getting into too much details, ketones may be in the form of acetoacetate, beta-hydroxybutyrate and acetone. Most likely, it is the acetone form that is causing your bad breath. So, how do you address this issue?

- Drink water often to help to remove bacteria from your mouth
- Use normal oral hygiene of brushing your teeth and use a good anti-bacterial mouthwash in the morning and evening.
- If you find yourself consuming excessive protein above the Keto Diet ranges of about 25 percent of your daily calories, reduce the amount of protein.
- Slightly increase your calories from carbohydrates (not too appealing if your come this far on the Keto Diet but still an option)

Once your body adjusts after a few weeks, your see this bad breath condition go away so you could decide to work through it on its own.

Risks and Side Effects to Consider – Constipation Due to a Change in Foods Being Consumed

Due to the elimination of numerous grains, fruits and vegetables, constipation will become a problem if not enough dietary fiber is obtained through the recommended Keto Diet vegetables.

- An option is to use fiber supplement tablets or powders (typically made from psyllium or methylcellulose) added to your meals for additional dietary fiber needs.
- There are also Ketogenic Diet specific fiber supplements available online or through specialty retailers.

Risks and Side Effects to Consider – Low Blood Sugar

If you are starting the Keto Diet from a high carbohydrate diet, low blood sugar (also known as hypoglycemia) is a common side effect as your body begins to use fat. Those who have been diagnosed as having insulin resistance or considered to be pre-diabetes or have diabetes due to an excess of carbohydrates in their diet will be affected the most.

- At the start of your Keto Diet, it is recommended to have fast acting glucose drinks or tablets available until your body has adjusted away from a high carbohydrate diet.
- However, if you suspect you may be pre-diabetes or diagnosed as pre-diabetes or have diabetes, please see your medical doctor or professional before starting the Keto Diet or any other diet without exception.

Risks and Side Effects to Consider – Vitamin and Nutrient Deficiencies

We reviewed earlier the importance of Micronutrients in your body needs daily. Because excess water will be flushed out of your body, be aware that there could be some mineral and electrolyte deficiencies you are experiencing including symptoms from the "Keto Flu".

- At a minimum, you should consider *taking a good natural multi-vitamin with minerals daily* which is what I do.
- I also recommend that you eat a sufficient amount of green vegetables high in potassium and other key minerals and vitamins, avocados (also has lots of healthy fats), nuts (moderate amounts) and low sugar fruit such as blackberries, raspberries and strawberries.

Risks and Side Effects to Consider – Heart Health

There have not been any long-term studies on the effect of eating a high amount of fat and protein from animal sources. This is in part because many individuals do not stay on a particular diet long enough as they are likely to cycle on and off with diets which can also be harmful to your metabolism.

However, it is essential to eat high quality proteins (for example, grass fed beef, pasture-raised animals, wild-caught seafood, limit or do not eat processed meats unless they are uncured, etc.) and high quality fats along with clean vegetables with sufficient fiber and nutrition.

Chapter 4: What is the Instant Pot

Describing the Instant Pot is somewhat difficult since it is useful for so many things. It is a multi-functional cooker. Just one pot can perform the job of several appliances. There are several different models available and some have more features than others. However, it is multifunctional and can perform a variety of tasks.

Depending on the model purchased, it can be used as a slow cooker, pressure cooker, rice cooker, Dutch oven, and that's just the beginning. Sautee' or steam veggies, or brown meat. Some models also have a yogurt making feature. If you are looking for the perfect all-in-one cooker, this is it.

Using the Instant Pot for a Slow Cooker

Slow cookers or crock pots have been popular for years because you can toss in a few ingredients, walk away and come home to supper. The instant pot is just a little more than a crock pot. For instance, it is designed with a microprocessor that can adjust heat levels, so you'll get consistent results. Another feature that enhances the slow cooker is the 24-hour timer. It can be used to make sure food is kept warm until you're ready to serve it. These features make it a good option for large batches of food.

Using it for a Pressure Cooker

The pressure cooker feature of the instant pot is probably one of the best-known functions of this handy device. Many people have been afraid of using a pressure cooker in the past, and some still are. It only takes one accident with the steam valve or blown off lid to earn your respect. This is why many people shy away from the traditional pressure cooking method. Thankfully, pressure cooking has evolved, and the Instant Pot can help remove the elements of guesswork and fear. It's about as easy as it gets. You select the setting and forget about it for a bit. You don't have to stand over the stove adjusting and readjusting the heat to make sure the pressure doesn't go too high or drop too low. This modern convenience lets you cook perfect creamy beans straight from the dried state without any presoaking. Or make hard-boiled eggs or baked potatoes in a matter of a few minutes. The pot has built-in features to indicate when the lid is locked safely and wen it's safe to open it again.

Cooking Grains in the Instant Pot

If your instant pot has the grains or rice feature, you can make a bowl of rice or oatmeal quickly and easily.

It's Just a Cooking Pot

The Instant Pot is also good for lots of general cooking jobs. Sautee' peppers and onions, steam veggies, or use it for browning meat. It's generally best to brown meat before cooking it anyway. Using the Instant Pot helps reduce the number of pans you have to cleanup later.

Use it for Baking

You can bake a wide variety of desserts in the Instant Pot. For your next get together you can bake up a cheesecake, custard, pudding, fruit cobbler or bread pudding. Some like to use it to bake quick breads.

Try it for Making Yogurt

If your IP includes the feature, you can even use it to make yogurt.

Chapter 5: Benefits of Using the Instant Pot

For each person who uses an Instant Pot for meal preparation, the specific benefits can vary. However, there are many advantages to using an Instant Pot. There are benefits you'll realize from using a pressure cooker specifically. Combine those benefits with the other features and you have a winning combination of lots of advantages. You can probably come up with a list of your own advantages, but let's look at a few of the prominent benefits most enjoy from using the IP.

Saving Time and Energy

Pressure cooking is a much faster method for cooking foods safely. For the most part, an electric pressure cooker reduces cooking time by as much as 70% over other cooking methods. The pot itself, uses less energy since there isn't as much water used in the cooking process. With a fully insulated external pot, not as much water is necessary. Electric pressure cookers are ranked as second when it comes to energy efficient cooking appliances, that's just behind microwaves.

PreNumber of Servings Nutrients

Pressure cooking delivers an even, deep heat and distributes it quickly. This is the reason you do not have to fully immerse food in water, you just need enough to create some steam to build up the pressure. Since the food is not submerged in water, the nutrients do not seep out of the food into the water. Steam surrounds food which means they do not become oxidized because of exposure air. If you notice, bright green veggies like broccoli retain those colors after cooking. The cooked food retains the original flavor. You may also notice while the IP is cooking, there is no smell of food wafting through the house. This is because the pot is sealed and holding in the nutrients.

Eliminate Dangerous Micro-Organisms

Pressure cookers use temperatures above the boiling point. This is high enough to kill most of the harmful micro-organisms like viruses and bacteria. A pressure cooker can also be used to sterilize jam pots and glass baby bottles. They've also been used to treat water. Some of the latest Instant Pots have a "sterilize' button for this purpose.

Many foods like corn, beans and rice are carriers for aflatoxins, or fungal poisons. The occur naturally in foods, usually because of improper storage practices. Humid conditions can encourage the growth of fungi. Aflatoxins have been known to trigger liver cancer and may possibly contribute to other types of cancers too. Heating food to the boiling point does not kill aflatoxins. Recent studies have indicated that pressure cooking does reduce the concentration of aflatoxins to a safe level.

Specific Instant Pot Benefits

Pressure cooking itself obviously has some advantages including health related ones. Here are a few of the benefits you will find as you venture into the world of the instant Pot.

Convenience

Depending on the model you invest in, you'll find anywhere from 5 or 6 single-key operation buttons to 12. These include a variety of common cooking tasks. These are as simple as placing the food in the pot, sealing it and pushing a button. Here are a few of the buttons you'll find convenient:

- Rice (white and multigrain settings)
- Porridge
- Sautee' or browning
- Soup
- Meat and stew

- Beans/chili
- Poultry
- Steaming
- Slow cook (old fashioned crock pot feature)
- Keep warm
- Yogurt

All the single button operation keys were designed specifically to help you achieve consistent results with your cooking. The manual pressure cooking button can be used, hence you can set the time your own recipes are cooked under pressure.

Programming

The on-button keys are pre-programed based on literally thousands of cooking experiments. They are pre-set to help you achieve the best result with your cooking ventures. Each button can also be refined to vary the taste from rare, normal or well done as per your family's preference.

Automatic Cooking

IP provides a lot of convenience by automating the cooking process. Each task is appropriately times and then automatically switches to the "keep warm" setting once cooking has completed. Conventional pressure cookers there isn't a timer, or food monitoring. You must manually keep the time and adjust the heat and length of time foods cook under pressure manually.

Delayed Cooking Feature

Just for a little more convenience, you can use the IP to delay cooking time up to 24 hours. This allows you to plan meals ahead of time. You are not required to stand over the stove and monitor your food's cooking. You don't even have to be in the kitchen. Load your food, set the delay timer to come on when you want it to and walk away. The delayed timer will cook your food and have it ready when you need it.

Trapped in Flavor

You already read how the pressure cooker seals in nutrients. However, the same process also seals in the flavor of your favorite, and not so favorite, foods. The pot is completely sealed which means the nutrients and aroma both stay in the pot, and in the food rather than being spread around the house. Fish, meat, fruits and veggies all retain their original juice and you'll enjoy the flavorful benefits.

Tasty and Tender

The IP cooks up meat and bones and makes them tender. When the cooking time has completed, the bones will separate from the tender meat. While cooking under pressure, whole grains and beans are softer and more flavorful than when they are cooked using other methods.

Energy Efficient

The Instant Pot is considered a "green" appliance because it saves as much as 70% electricity when compared to other cooking appliances. There is a good reason the Instant Pot cooks so efficiently. It was designed that way. There features ensure the IP works efficiently.

- Food cooks faster when it is under pressure and high temperature. Less cooking time equates to consuming less energy.
- The exterior portion of the IP is fully insulated. It's made up of two layers of air pockets situated between the inner pot and the outside of the pot. It's cool to touch and gets only lukewarm when it cooks for long periods of time.

- The IP has an intelligent monitoring system. This means it only heats to a certain pressure level. When cooking something for a long time, heating will be off about 40% of the total cooking time.

- The unique sealing feature of the IP requires less water to be used. This reduces the heat the IP puts off, which means your kitchen doesn't get all hot and steamy when cooking during the summer months.

Unique Safety Features

Conventional stove-top pressure cooker disasters were because of user error. However, the new Instant Pot is designed so that most potential problems are avoided or eliminated altogether. Instant Pot is manufactured by the leading manufacturer of pressure cookers. They have already put 10 million in households around the globe.

Stove-top pressure cookers use a weighted regulator on the lid to help maintain pressure. The Instant Pot uses a patented sensor which is more precise and automated. When the inside pressure builds, the bottom of the pot, called the flat, flexible board, shifts downward and triggers the pressure sensor. It moves back up as the pressure releases. The sensor controls the heating element to help keep the pressure inside a safe range.

There are 10 safety features built in to the Instant Pot.

1 Lid Close Detection – if the lid is not properly closed, the functions will not work.

2 Leaky Lid Protection – if the cooker lid leaks, the cooker will not function. It will not heat to the pre-set pressure level. The pot can sense when the pre-heating time is not right. If it takes too long to heat up, the pot will switch to keep warm, so

food doesn't burn.

3 - Lid-Lock – The lid will remain locked as long as the cooker is holding pressure.

4 - Vent for Anti-blockage – When food is cooking, it could jam the steam release vent. There is a special shield protecting the vent from becoming blocked.

5 - Temperature Control – A built-in thermostat regulates the temperature of the inner pot to ensure it stays in a safe range for the foods being cooked.

6 - High Temp Warnings – Pressure will not operate if there is no water or moisture inside. To avoid overheating, the IP will stop heating after the temp reaches a certain limit.

7 - Power Shut-off – If the pot reaches too high of a temperature, it will shut off automatically.

8 - Automated Pressure Controls - A sensor mechanism keeps the pressure at the right psi.

9 - Regulating Pressure – If the pressure exceeds 15.23 psi, it will automatically start to release steam to bring down the pressure in the pot.

10 - Excessive Pressure – If the pressure reaches an extreme level and the pressure regulator fails to function, it will activate the internal protection mechanism. This creates a gap between the lid and inner pot to which steam is released. This stops the heating and releases pressure.

Chapter 6: Breakfast Recipes

Breakfast Mexican Omelet

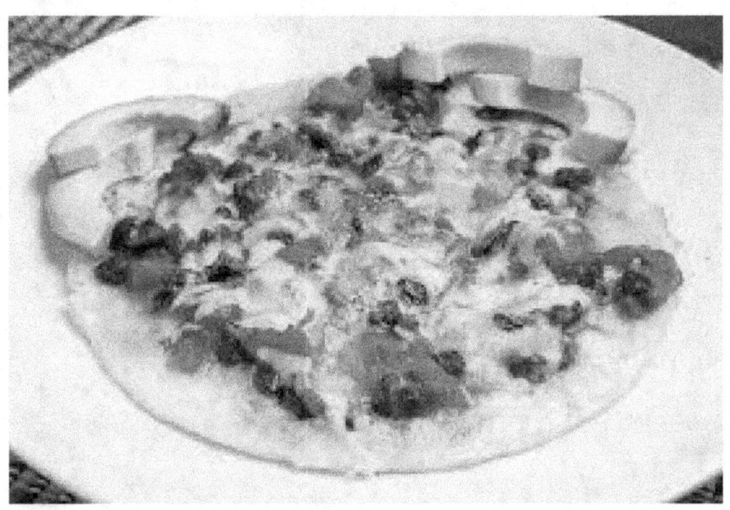

Prep time: 4 minutes

Cook time: 9 minutes

Number of Servings: 1

Ingredients

- ½ tablespoon lime juice

- 2 eggs 1 tablespoon water

- 1 tablespoon crumbled bacon

- 1/2 tablespoon butter

- ¼ avocado

- ½ cup hand-shredded Mexican cheese

- 2 tablespoon Pace Thick and Chunky Medium Salsa

Directions

1. Melt the butter in a microwaveable bowl in the microwave.

2. Quickly whip the wet ingredients in a microwaveable bowl, can be the same bowl as before.

3. Microwave for one minute.

4. Place on warm plate.

5. Top with all the rest of the ingredients.

6. Combine the wet ingredients in a zip-lock bag, except the butter and water. Refrigerate. Combine the water and butter in a zip-lock bag.

Nutritional Value:

Calories: 275,

Total Fat: 21,

Protein: 17g,

Total Carbs: 3.2g,

Dietary Fiber: 2g,

Sugar: 2g,

Sodium: 230mg

Breakfast Casserole

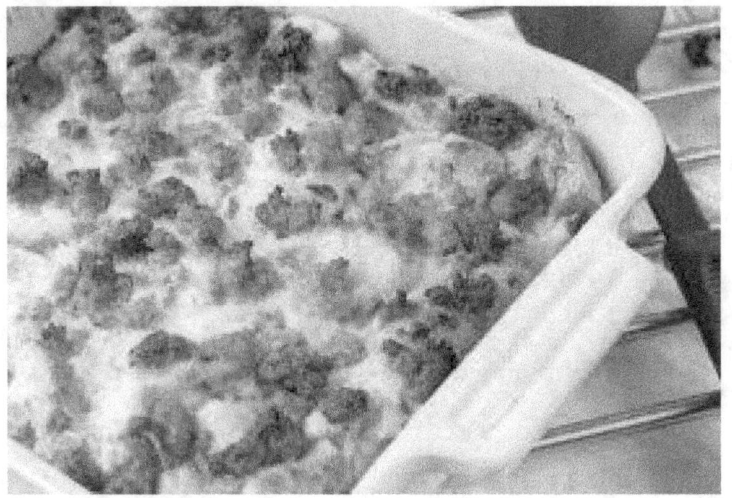

Prep time: 4 minutes

Cook time: 19 minutes

Number of Servings: 4

Ingredients

- 8 oz Sausage, Cooked and Crumbled

- 1 cup hot salsa

- 4 eggs

- 2 chopped green onions

- ¼ cup hand-shredded pepper jack or cheddar cheese

- ½ bell pepper, chopped, your choice of color

Directions

1. Place oven rack to the middle shelf setting.

2. Heat oven to 400 degrees.

3. Cook the peppers until soft.

4. Spray or grease the baking dishes excessively. Eggs stick when baked.

5. Layer ingredients in 4 individual baking dishes, like Corning ware "grab-its," any bakeware that holds one cup servings.

6. Layer with sausage first, then peppers, then cheese.

7. Add one whipped egg to each baking dish. Sprinkle with green onions.

8. Bake for 18 minutes, until eggs are set.

9. Place cooled casseroles in individual freezer bags. Reheat in microwave for 2-3 minutes until hot.

Nutritional Value:

Calories: 195,

Total Fat: 11g,

Protein: 19g,

Total Carbs: 3g,

Dietary Fiber: 1g,

Sugar: 0,

Sodium: 112mg

Cinnamon Chocolate Smoothie

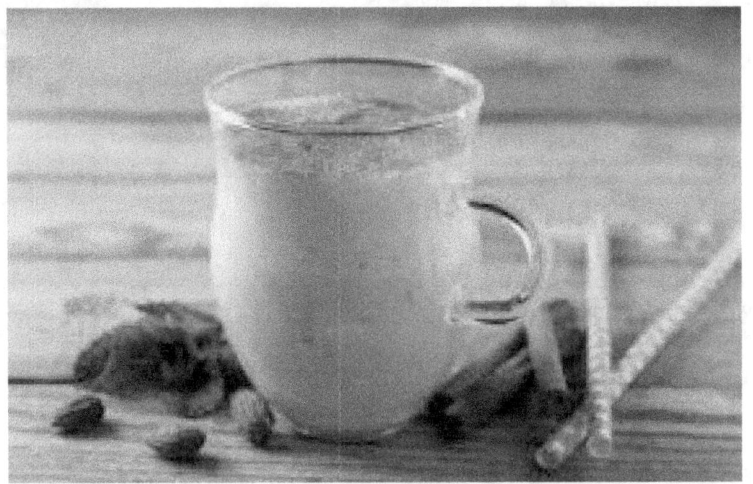

Prep time: 4 minutes

Cook time: 0 minutes

Number of Servings: 1

Ingredients

- ½ cup firm Tofu
- 2 tablespoon cocoa powder
- 1 scoop chocolate protein powder
- 2 tablespoon cinnamon
- 2 sweetener packets
- 1 cup almond milk, unsweetened
- 4 ice cubes

Directions

1. Place all the ingredients in a blender, pulse until desired consistency, and serve.

2. Refrigerate the tofu. Place all the dry ingredients into one snack sized zip-lock bag.

Nutritional Value:

Calories: 273,

Total Fat: 15g,

Protein: 33g,

Total Carbs: 9g,

Dietary Fiber: 20g,

Sugar: 2g,

Sodium: 214mg

Black and Blue Smoothie

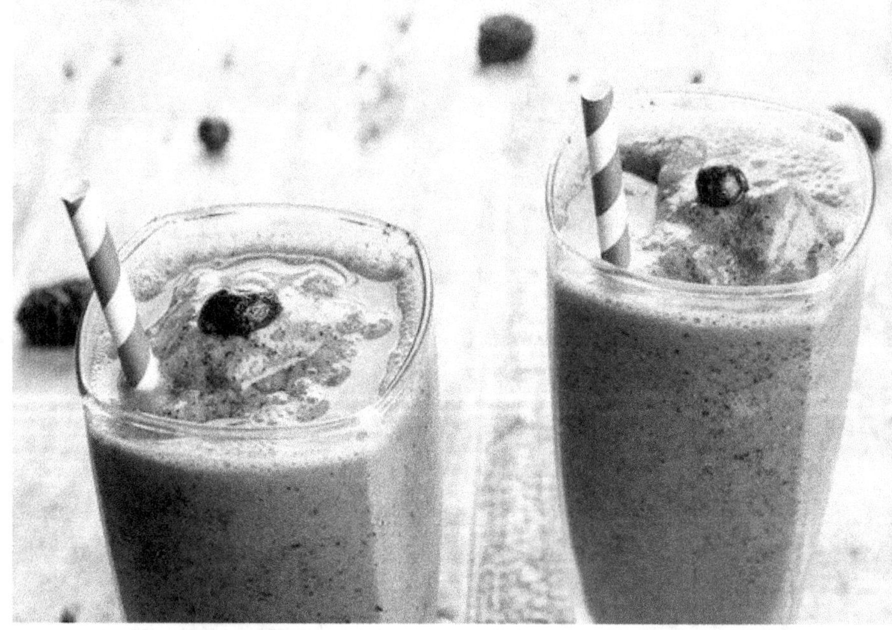

Prep time: 4 minutes

Cook time: 0 minutes

Number of Servings: 1

Ingredients

- ¼ cup Frozen Blueberries

- ¼ cup Frozen Blackberries

- 1 cup unsweetened soy or almond milk

- 1 tablespoon vanilla

- 1 scoop (your choice) vanilla whey protein powder

- 2 packets sweetener of your choice

- 3 tablespoon flaxseeds

Directions

1. Mix the ingredients and emulsify by blending.

2. Pulse four times or until desired thickness.

3. Pour into a glass and enjoy.

4. Combine berries in freezer bags and place in the freezer. Combine sweetener of your choice, flaxseeds, and protein powder in zip-lock bags. Combine milk and vanilla in 1 cup containers in the fridge.

Nutritional Value:

Calories: 221,

Total Fat: 9.8g,

Protein: 21.8g,

Total Carbs: 10g,

Dietary Fiber: 5.8g,

Sugar: 1g,

Sodium: 0mg

Cheese Blintz with Blueberries

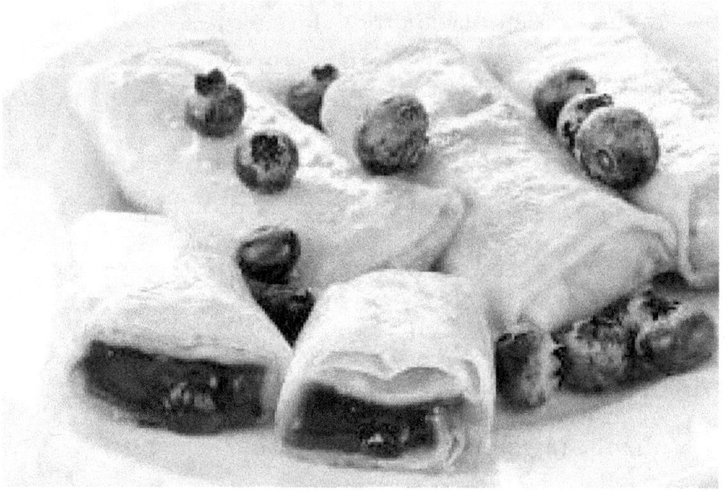

Prep time: 9 minutes

Cook time: 4 minutes

Number of Servings: 1

Ingredients

- 1 medium egg

- 1 tablespoon half & half

- 1 scoop protein shake powder, vanilla

- 1 pat of butter

- 1 tablespoon of olive oil

- 2 tablespoon ricotta cheese

- 1 tablespoon Greek yogurt, plain

- 1 packet sweetener

- 1 tablespoon cinnamon

- ½ cup blueberries

Directions

1. Combine the ricotta cheese, Greek yogurt, sweetener and cinnamon in a bowl, mix well.

2. Combine the egg, protein powder, and cream. Whisk until all lumps are dissolved, and the mixture is well-blended.

3. Coat a non-stick skillet with the olive oil.

4. At medium heat, melt butter in the skillet and pour the batter on top.

5. Swirl the skillet until the batter is evenly distributed. When the batter has set, gently turn the blintz to the other side.

6. Let cook for one minute until the batter is set, but not browned.

7. Gently fold half the blueberries into the filling.

8. Place the filling in the middle of the blitz.

9. Roll into a pancake and serve with the remaining blueberries.

10. Mix the filling and place in the fridge in a covered container. Place the blueberries in a zip-lock bag and place in the freezer.

Nutritional Value:

Calories: 427

Total Fat: 23g,

Protein: 39g,

Total Carbs: 14g,

Dietary Fiber: 3g,

Sugar: 10g,

Sodium: 330mg

Almond Joy Microwave Muffin

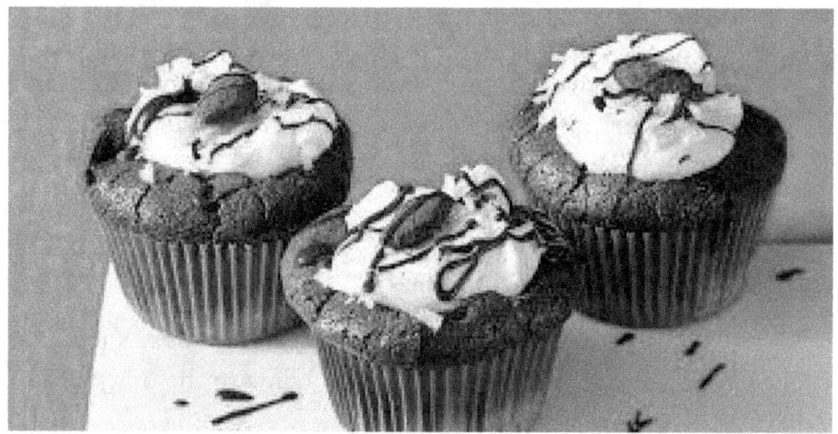

Prep time: 3 minutes

Cook time: 1 minutes

Number of Servings: 1

Ingredients

- 2 tablespoon almond flour

- 1 tablespoon Coconut Flour

- 1 packet Splenda

- 1/4 tablespoon Baking Powder

- Sprinkle with Salt

- 1 Egg

- 1 tablespoon butter

- 1 tablespoon cocoa

Directions

1. Combine the dry ingredients in a microwaveable mug.

2. Quickly whip the egg and the oil together.

3. Stir into the dry mixture.

4. Microwave on high for 1 minute.

5. Toast with butter.

6. Place all dry ingredients in zip-lock baggies, 1 recipe per bag. Do not premix the eggs and oil. Wait until morning for combining.

Nutritional Value:

Calories: 207,

Total Fat: 16.8g,

Protein: 9.7g,

Total Carbs: 3.7g,

Dietary Fiber: 3,

Sugar: 0,

Sodium: 300mg

Butter Pecan Waffles

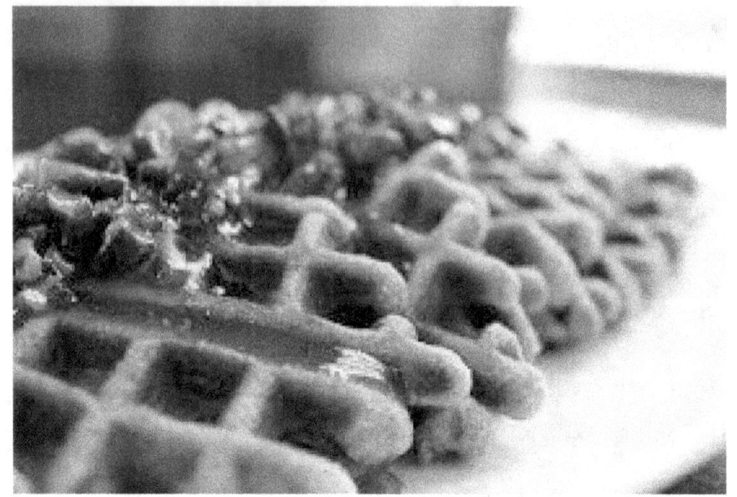

Prep time: 9 minutes

Cook time: 4 minutes

Number of Servings: 4

Ingredients

- 1 cup soy flour

- 2 packets Splenda

- 3 tablespoon baking powder

- ¾ cup buttermilk

- 1 tablespoon butter

- ½ tablespoon baking soda

- 3 eggs

- 2 tablespoon vanilla

- ½ cup water

- 2 tablespoon sugar free butter rum flavoring

- ½ cup pecans

Directions

1. Combine everything except the pecans.

2. Use ¼ c batter for cooking the waffle.

3. Cook until crisp.

4. Top with pecans and sugar free syrup.

5. After the waffle is cool, place 1 per zip-lock bag. Warm by toasting in the toaster.

Nutritional Value:

Calories: 181,

Total Fat: 13g,

Protein: 9g,

Total Carbs: 5g,

Dietary Fiber: 2g,

Sugar: 3g,

Sodium: 178mg

Kale Wrapped Eggs

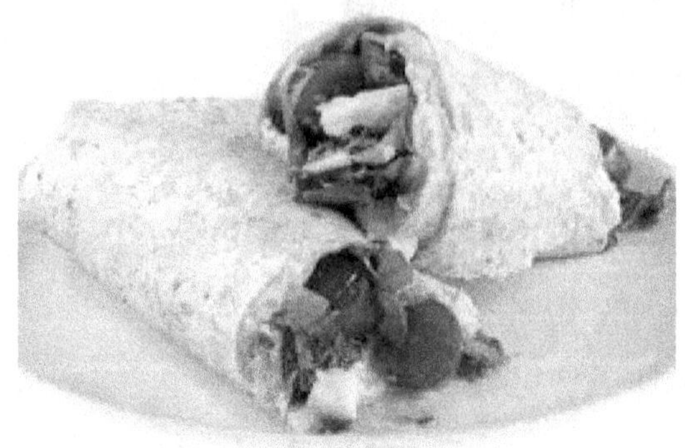

Prep Time: 8-10 min.

Cooking Time: 5 min.

Number of Servings: 4

Ingredients:

- 3 tablespoons heavy cream
- 4 hardboiled eggs
- ¼ teaspoon pepper
- 4 kale leaves
- 4 prosciutto slices
- ¼ teaspoon salt
- 1 ½ cups water

Directions:

1. Peel the eggs and wrap each with the kale. Wrap them in the prosciutto slices and sprinkle with ground black pepper and salt.

2. Arrange Instant Pot over a dry platform in your kitchen. Open its top lid and switch it on.

3. In the pot, pour water. Arrange a trivet or steamer basket inside that came with Instant Pot. Now place/arrange the eggs over the trivet/basket.

4. Close top lid to create a locked chamber; make sure that safety valve is in locking position.

5. Find and press "MANUAL" cooking function; timer to 5 minutes with default "HIGH" pressure mode.

6. Allow the pressure to build to cook the ingredients.

7. After cooking time is over, press "CANCEL" setting. Find and press "QPR" cooking function. This setting is for quick release of inside pressure.

8. Slowly open the lid, take out the cooked recipe in serving plates or serving bowls and enjoy the keto recipe.

Nutritional Values (Per Serving):

Calories - 247

Fat – 20g

Saturated Fat – 6g

Trans Fat – 0g

Carbohydrates – 7g

Fiber – 3g

Sodium – 742mg

Protein – 19g

Zucchini Keto Bread

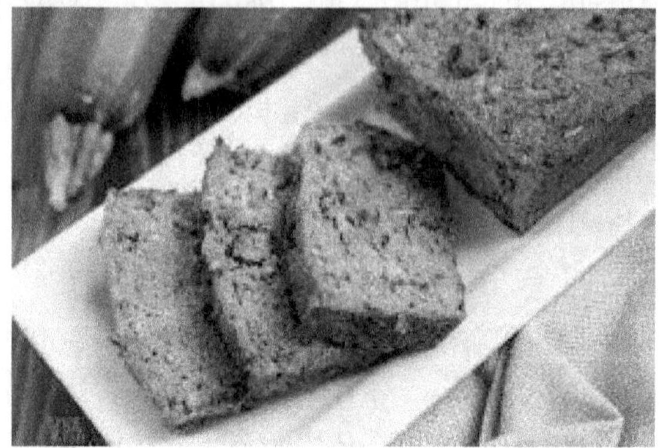

Prep Time: 8-10 min.

Cooking Time: 40 min.

Number of Servings: 12-16 slices

Ingredients:

- 1 cup grated zucchini
- 2 ½ cups almond flour
- ½ cup chopped walnuts
- 3 eggs
- ½ cup olive oil
- 1 ½ teaspoon baking powder
- Pinch of ginger powder
- 1 teaspoon vanilla extract
- ½ teaspoon cinnamon
- ¼ teaspoon nutmeg
- pinch of sea salt
- 1 ½ cups water

Directions:

1. Whisk together the wet ingredients in a bowl.

2. Combine the dry ingredients in another bowl. Combine the dry and wet mixture together. Stir in the zucchini.

3. Grease a loaf pan with some butter and pour the mixture. Top with chopped walnuts.

4. Arrange Instant Pot over a dry platform in your kitchen. Open its top lid and switch it on.

5. In the pot, pour water. Arrange a trivet or steamer basket inside that came with Instant Pot. Now place/arrange the loaf pan over the trivet/basket.

6. Close top lid to create a locked chamber; make sure that safety valve is in locking position.

7. Find and press "MANUAL" cooking function; timer to 40 minutes with default "HIGH" pressure mode.

8. Allow the pressure to build to cook the ingredients.

9. After cooking time is over, press "CANCEL" setting. Find and press "QPR" cooking function. This setting is for quick release of inside pressure.

10. Slowly open the lid, take out the cooked bread.

11. Cool down; slice and serve.

Nutritional Values (Per Serving):

Calories – 164

Fat – 17g

Saturated Fat – 2g

Trans Fat – 0g

Carbohydrates – 3g

Fiber – 2g

Sodium – 94mg

Protein – 5g

Ham Sausage Quiche

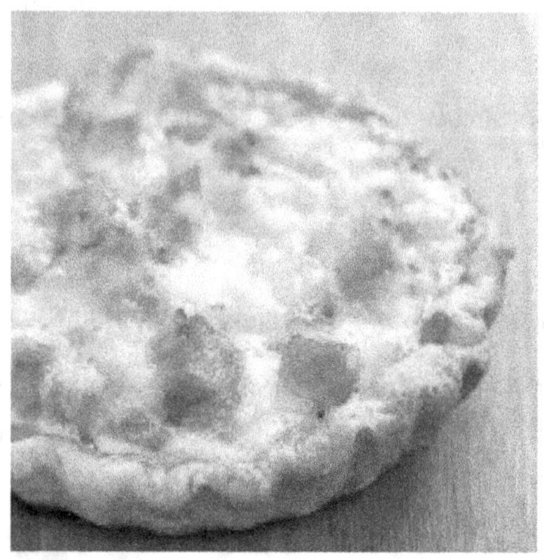

Prep Time: 8-10 min.

Cooking Time: 30 min.

Number of Servings: 4

Ingredients:

- 4 bacon slices, cooked and crumbled

- ½ cup diced ham

- 2 green onions, chopped

- ½ cup full-fat milk

- 6 eggs, beaten

- 1 cup ground sausage, cooked

- 1 cup shredded cheddar cheese

- ¼ teaspoon salt

- Pinch of pepper

- 1 ½ cups water

Directions:

1. Grease a baking dish with coconut oil cooking spray.

2. Place all of the ingredients in a bowl, and stir to combine. Add this mixture to the prepared dish.

3. Arrange Instant Pot over a dry platform in your kitchen. Open its top lid and switch it on.

4. In the pot, pour water. Arrange a trivet or steamer basket inside that came with Instant Pot. Now place/arrange the dish over the trivet/basket.

5. Close top lid to create a locked chamber; make sure that safety valve is in locking position.

6. Find and press "MANUAL" cooking function; timer to 30 minutes with default "HIGH" pressure mode.

7. Allow the pressure to build to cook the ingredients.

8. After cooking time is over, press "CANCEL" setting. Find and press "QPR" cooking function. This setting is for quick release of inside pressure.

9. Place the dish on the rack in your IP and close the lid. Cook on HIGH for 30 minutes. Release the pressure naturally, for 10 minutes.

10. Slowly open the lid, take out the cooked recipe in serving plates or serving bowls and enjoy the keto recipe.

Nutritional Values (Per Serving):

Calories - 398

Fat – 31g

Saturated Fat – 13g

Trans Fat – 0g

Carbohydrates – 5g

Fiber – 1g

Sodium – 745mg

Protein – 26g

Coconut Almond Breakfast

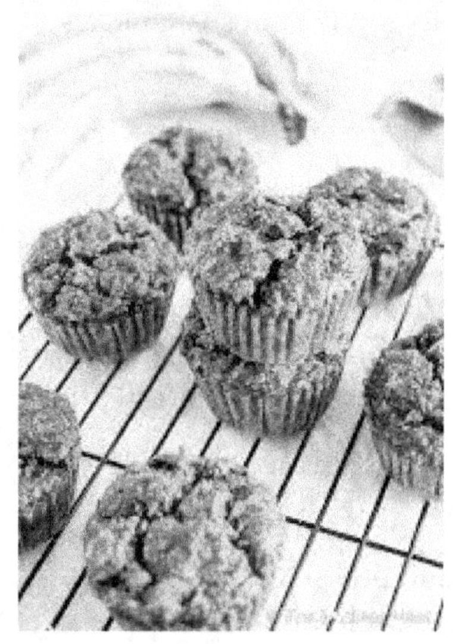

Prep Time: 8-10 min.

Cooking Time: 5 min.

Number of Servings: 2

Ingredients:

- 2 tablespoons roasted pepitas

- 1/3 cup coconut milk

- 2 tablespoon chopped almonds

- 1 tablespoon chia seeds

- 1/3 cup water

- One handful blueberries

Directions:

1. In your food processor or blender, mix the pepitas with almonds and pulse them well.

2. Arrange Instant Pot over a dry platform in your kitchen. Open its top lid and switch it on.

3. Add the chia seeds with water and coconut milk; gently stir to mix well.

4. Add the pepita mix and combine.

5. Close top lid to create a locked chamber; make sure that safety valve is in locking position.

6. Find and press "MANUAL" cooking function; timer to 5 minutes with default "HIGH" pressure mode.

7. Allow the pressure to build to cook the ingredients.

8. After cooking time is over, press "CANCEL" setting. Find and press "QPR" cooking function. This setting is for quick release of inside pressure.

9. Slowly open the lid, take out the cooked recipe in serving plates or serving bowls, top with the blueberries, and enjoy the keto recipe.

Nutritional Values (Per Serving):

Calories - 148

Fat – 6g

Saturated Fat – 1g

Trans Fat – 0g

Carbohydrates – 4g

Fiber – 2g

Sodium – 346mg

Protein – 2g

Avocado Egg Muffins

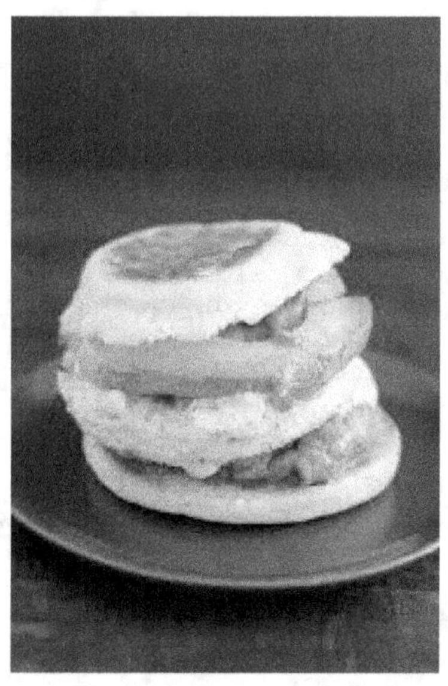

Prep Time: 8-10 min.

Cooking Time: 12 min.

Number of Servings: 4

Ingredients:

- 1 ½ cups coconut milk

- 2 avocados, diced

- 4 ½ ounces (grated or shredded) cheese

- ½ cup almond flour

- 5 bacon slices, cooked and crumbled

- 5 eggs, beaten

- 2 tablespoon butter

- 3 spring onions, diced

- 1 teaspoon oregano

- ¼ cup flaxseed meal

- 1 ½ tablespoon lemon juice

- 1 teaspoon minced garlic

- 1 teaspoon onion powder

- 1 teaspoon salt

- Pinch of pepper

- 1 teaspoon baking powder

- 1 ½ cups water

Directions:

1. Whisk together the wet ingredients.

2. Gradually stir in the dry ingredients; mix until turns smooth. Stir in the avocado, bacon, onions, and cheese.

3. Add the mixture into 16 muffin cups.

4. Arrange Instant Pot over a dry platform in your kitchen. Open its top lid and switch it on.

5. In the pot, pour water. Arrange a trivet or steamer basket inside that came with Instant Pot. Now place/arrange the 8 cups over the trivet/basket.

6. Close top lid to create a locked chamber; make sure that safety valve is in locking position.

7. Find and press "MANUAL" cooking function; timer to 12 minutes with default "HIGH" pressure mode.

8. Allow the pressure to build to cook the ingredients.

9. After cooking time is over, press "CANCEL" setting. Find and press "QPR" cooking function. This setting is for quick release of inside pressure.

10. Slowly open the lid, take out the cooked recipe in serving plates or serving bowls and enjoy the keto recipe.

11. Repeat the same process.

Nutritional Values (Per Serving):

Calories - 146

Fat – 11g

Saturated Fat – 3g

Trans Fat – 0g

Carbohydrates – 4g

Fiber – 2g

Sodium – 356mg

Protein – 6g

Chapter 7: Lunch

Chicken Lettuce Wraps

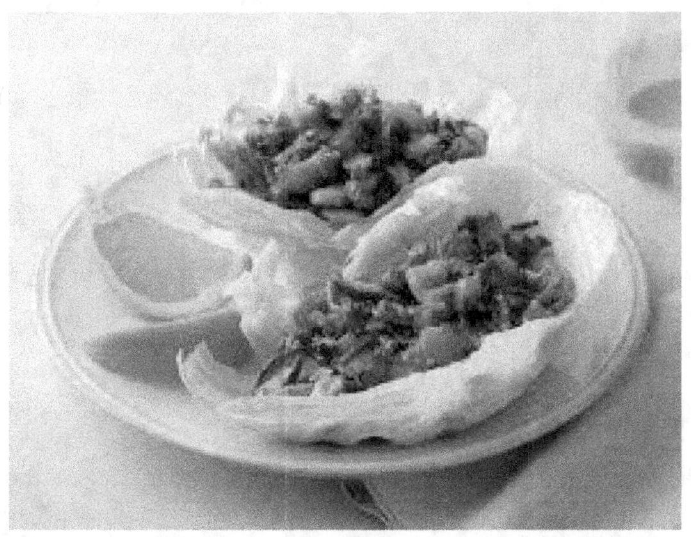

Prep time: 10minutes

Cook time: 10minutes

Number of Servings: 1

Ingredients

- 1 chicken breast, boneless, diced into 1-inch size pieces

- 1 cup diced or sliced fresh mushrooms

- ½ cup diced water chestnuts (from a can, drained)

- 1 tablespoon olive oil

- 1 tablespoon onion, minced

- 1 tablespoon minced garlic

- 1 tablespoon teriyaki sauce

- garlic powder, only a dash

- onion powder, just a dash

- oregano, one dash

- cayenne pepper, a small dash

- salt /pepper

Directions

1. Mix the ingredients and cook in a skillet until the chicken is done, about 10 minutes.

2. Shred the chicken

3. Place in leaves and roll

4. Place all ingredients into one freezer bag except the lettuce. Microwave one minute and serve.

Nutritional Value:

Calories: 145,

Total Fat: 1g,

Protein: 35g,

Dietary Fiber: 1g,

Total Carbs: 4g,

Sugar: 0g,

Sodium: 100mg

Indian Chicken Curry

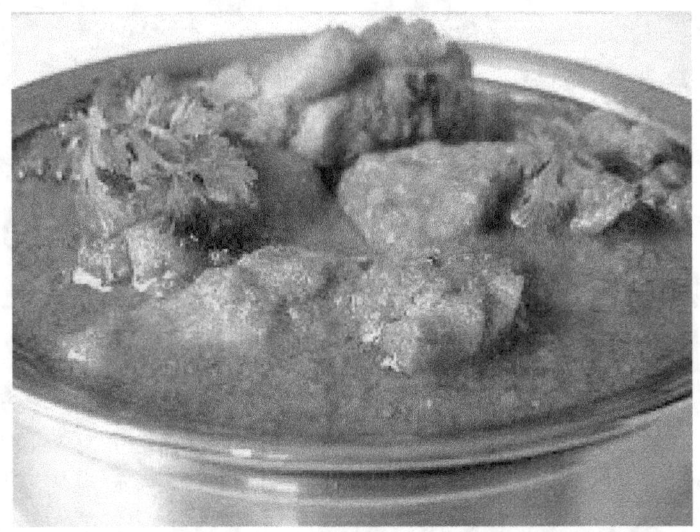

Prep Time: 2 Hours

Number of Servings: 4

Ingredients:

- 6 chicken thighs, cut into small pieces

- 1 onion, diced

- 4 cloves of garlic, minced

- 1 tablespoon of salt

- 2 tablespoon of red curry paste

- 2 tablespoon of curry, powdered

- 2 tablespoon of soy sauce

- 5 drops of Stevia

- 3 tablespoon of cilantro, fresh, chopped and extra for garnish

- ¼ cup of extra virgin olive oil

- 3 tablespoon of coconut oil

- ½ cup of heavy cream

- 2 tablespoon of cornstarch

- 2 tablespoon of cold water

- 1 lime, fresh and juice only

Directions:

1. Use a large bowl and add in the chicken thigh pieces, onion, garlic, dash of salt, red curry paste, powdered curry, soy sauce, stevia, cilantro and extra virgin olive oil. Stir well to mix.

2. Cover the bowl and set into the fridge to marinate for 1 hour.

3. After this time place a large skillet over medium to high heat. Add in the coconut oil and once the oil is hot enough add in the marinated chicken. Cook for 8 to 10 minutes or until the chicken is cooked through.

4. Pour in the coconut milk and bring the mixture to a boil. Once boiling reduce the heat to low. Cover and cook for 30 to 40 minutes. Make sure to stir the chicken every 5 to 10 minutes.

5. Add in the heavy cream after this time and increase the heat to high. Bring the mixture to a boil.

6. While the mixture is coming to a boil add the cornstarch and water into a small bowl. Whisk to make a slurry and pour into the chicken mixture. Stir well to mix and cook for 5 minutes or until thick in consistency.

7. Add in the fresh lime juice and a dash of salt.

8.   Remove from heat and serve.

Nutritional Value:

Calories: 408,

Fat: 32 grams,

Carbs: 7 grams,

Protein: 23 grams

No Bake Cheesecake

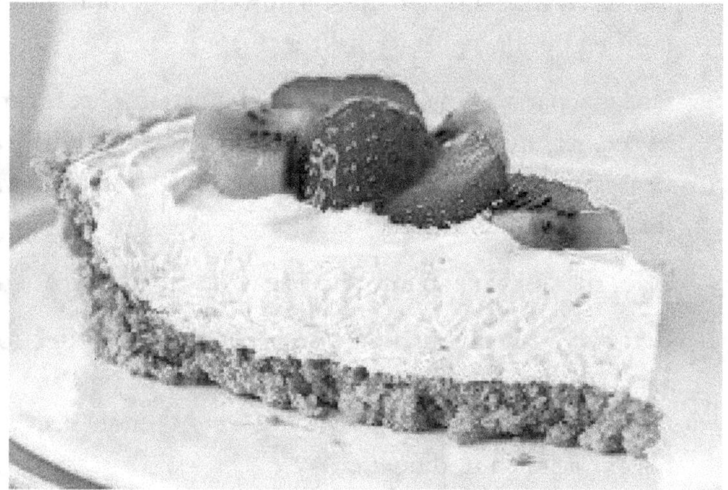

Prep Time: 6 Hours and 15 Minutes

Number of Servings: 4

Ingredients:

- ½ cup of almond flour

- ¼ cup of butter, melted

- 16 ounces of cream cheese, soft

- ¾ cup of artificial sweetener

- ½ tablespoon of pure vanilla

- ½ tablespoon of lemon juice, fresh

- ½ tablespoon of salt

Directions:

1. Spray a muffin pan with cooking spray and line with paper muffin lines.

2. Use a large bowl and add in the almond flour and butter. Stir well until mixed. Pour this mixture into the bottom of each muffin cup. Press flat to make a crust.

3. Use a separate bowl and add in the cream cheese, artificial sweetener, pure vanilla, fresh lemon juice and dash of salt. Beat with an electric mixer until creamy in consistency. Pour this mixture over the crusts.

4. Place the muffin pan into the freezer to freeze for 2 hours.

5. Remove after this time and transfer into the fridge to thaw for 3 to 4 hours. Serve. Flank Steak Stuffed with Pancetta and Goat Cheese This is a great tasting keto friendly dish you can make for lunch or dinner.

Nutritional Value:

Calories: 195,

Fat: 19 grams,

Carbs: 3 grams,

Protein: 3 grams

Italian Eggplant Lasagna

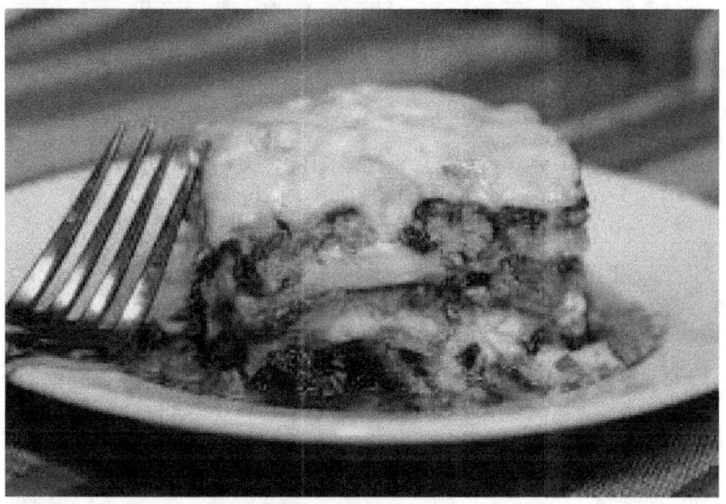

Prep time: 1 Hour and 45 Minutes

Number of Servings: 4

Ingredients:

- 1 eggplant, sliced thinly

- 2 tablespoon of salt

- 6 tablespoon of extra virgin olive oil

- 1 pound of Italian sausage

- 2 cups of ricotta cheese

- 2 cups of marinara sauce

- 3 cups of mozzarella cheese, shredded

- 2 cups of Parmesan cheese, grated

Directions:

1. Place the eggplant slices on a flat surface. Season with a dash of salt and set aside to sit for 20 to 30 minutes.

2. Preheat the oven to 400 degrees.

3. Pat dry the paper towels with a sheet of paper towels.

4. Drizzle the olive oil over the eggplant slices and place onto a large baking sheet. Place into the oven to roast for 10 minutes.

5. While the eggplant slices are roasting place a large skillet over medium heat. Add in the Italian sausage and cook for 10 to 12 minutes or until cooked through. Remove and set aside.

6. Reduce the temperature in the oven to 375 degrees.

7. Then use a large bowl and add in the Italian sausage and ricotta cheese. Stir well to mix. Pour half a cup of this mixture into the bottom of a large greased baking dish. Lay down 1/3 of the eggplant slices into the baking dish. Repeat the layers. Top off with the marinara sauce, mozzarella cheese and Parmesan cheese.

8. Cover the baking dish with a sheet of aluminum foil. Place into the oven to bake for 30 to 40 minutes. Remove the aluminum foil and continue to bake for another 10 minutes or until browned.

9. Remove from the oven and allow cooling for 20 minutes before serving.

Nutritional Value:

Calories: 667,

Fat: 51 grams,

Carbs: 14 grams,

Protein: 38 grams

Chicken Piccata

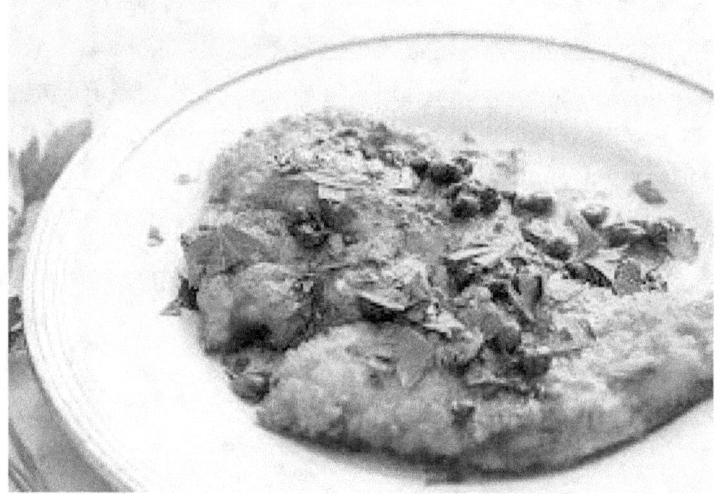

Prep time: 20 Minutes

Number of Servings: 4

Ingredients:

- 4 chicken thighs Dash of salt and black pepper

- 4 tablespoon of extra virgin olive oil

- 6 ounces of butter, soft

- ¼ cup of white wine, dried

- ¼ cup of lemon juice, fresh

- ½ cup of chicken stock

- ¼ cup of capers, brined

- 4 tablespoon of heavy cream

- ¼ cup of parsley, fresh and chopped

Directions:

1. Season the chicken thighs with a dash of salt and black pepper.

2. Place a large saucepan over medium to high heat. Add in the extra virgin olive oil and two tablespoons of soft butter. Once the butter begins to simmer add in the chicken thighs. Cook for 5 minutes on each side or until cooked through. Remove from the saucepan and transfer to a large plate.

3. Add the dried white wine into the saucepan and deglaze the pan.

4. Add in the fresh lemon juice, chicken stock and capers. Stir well to mix and bring the mixture to a boil. Once boiling reduces the heat to low.

5. Add the chicken back into the saucepan. Allow to simmer for 5 minutes.

6. Transfer the chicken back into a large plate.

7. Add the heavy cream and remaining butter into the saucepan. Season with a dash of salt and black pepper. Whisk to mix.

8. Pour the sauce over the chicken. Serve with a garnish of parsley.

Nutritional Value:

Calories: 468,

Fat: 39 grams,

Carbs: 3.6 grams,

Protein: 28 grams

Chili Mac

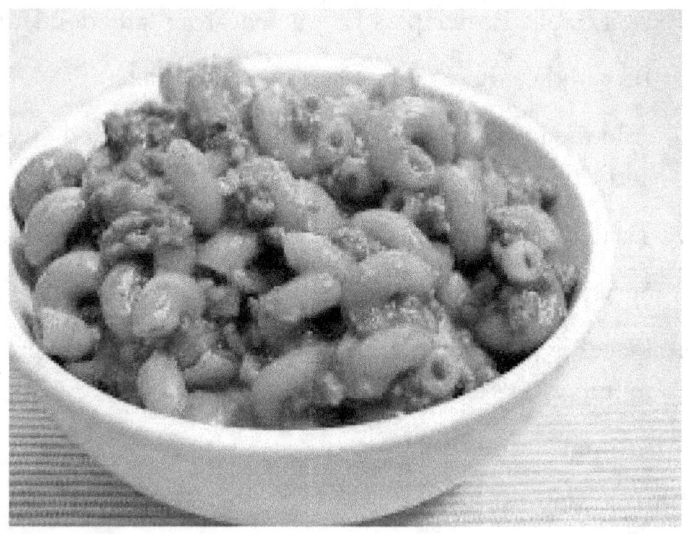

Prep time: 9 minutes

Cook time: 9 minutes

Number of Servings: 4

Ingredients

- 1 lb ground Sirloin

- 1 chopped Onion

- 1 Chili Seasoning Mix, packet

- 1 cup tomato sauce

- 1 small can of Chunky Diced Tomatoes & Green Chilies

- 1 cup hand-shredded sharp cheddar

- 1 packet Splenda

- ½ cup Barilla Proteinplus Elbow macaroni

Directions

1. Boil Barilla Proteinplus Elbow macaroni until done, drain.

2. Brown the sirloin and onions in a large skillet.

3. Add the pasta, tomato sauce, diced tomatoes and green chilies, and chili seasoning mix.

4. Taste to see if you need to add water.

5. Serve in 4 bowls, topping each bowl with the cheddar cheese.

6. Place in four containers with lids, freeze. Microwave 2 minutes to thaw.

Nutritional Value:

Calories: 480,

Total Fat: 24g,

Protein: 36g,

Total Carbs: 25g,

Dietary Fiber: 6g,

Sugar: 4g,

Sodium: 995mg

Stuffed with goat cheese,

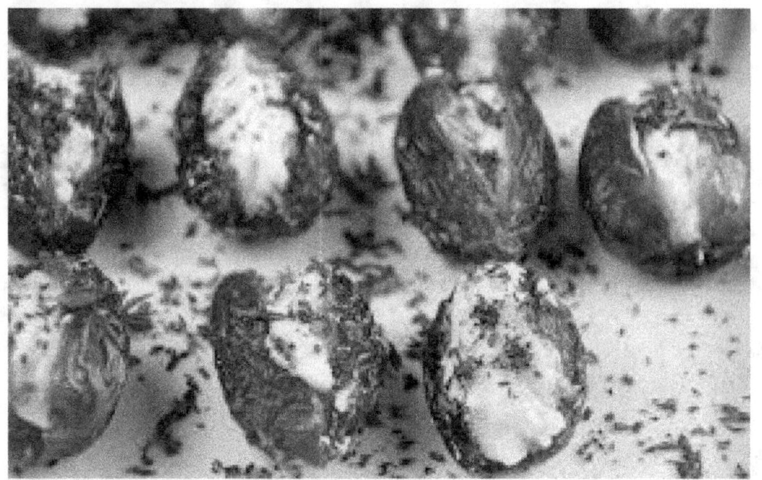

Prep Time: 5 Hours and 30 Minutes

Number of Servings: 4

Ingredients:

- ¼ cup of red wine

- ¼ cup of balsamic vinegar

- 2 tablespoon of Dijon mustard

- 2 tablespoon of soy sauce

- 1 cup of extra virgin olive oil

- 4 cloves of garlic, peeled and thinly sliced

- 1 tablespoon of salt Dash of black pepper

- 1, 2 to 3 pounds of flank steak

Ingredients for the stuffing:

- ½ cup of pancetta, cooked and chopped

- 8 ounces of goat cheese

- 3 cups of spinach, drained and excess liquid drained

Directions:

1. Use a large bowl and add in the red wine, vinegar, mustard, soy sauce, olive oil, garlic and dash of salt and black pepper. Whisk until mixed.

2. Add in the flank steak and cover. Set in the fridge to marinate for 4 hours.

3. Place a large saucepan over low heat. Chop the pancetta and place into the saucepan. Cook for 20 to 30 minutes. Drain the excess fat and set the pancetta aside.

4. Add the spinach into the saucepan and cook for 1 to 2 minutes or until fragrant. Remove from the pan and squeeze out the excess liquid. Add into a bowl with the pancetta and goat cheese. Stir well to mix.

5. Remove the flank steak from the marinade and place onto a flat surface. Beat with a meat mallet until ¼ inch in thickness.

6. Spread the stuffing onto the flank steak. Roll and tie with twine to seal. Season with a dash of salt and black pepper.

7. Heat up the oven to 400 degrees.

8. Place the rolled flank steak onto a large baking sheet and drizzle a few drops of olive oil over the top.

9. Place into the oven to bake for 15 to 25 minutes or until cooked through. Remove and allow to rest for 15 minutes before serving.

Nutritional Value:

Calories: 646,

Fat: 58 grams,

Carbs: 4 grams,

Protein: 27 grams

Mushroom Beef Chili

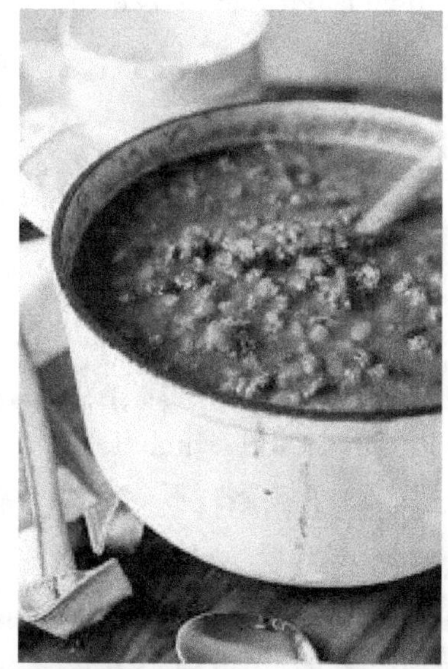

Prep Time: 8-10 min.

Cooking Time: 30 min.

Number of Servings: 4

Ingredients:

- 2 tablespoons (finely ground) cumin
- 1 tablespoon chili powder
- 1 tablespoon paprika
- 1 tablespoon olive oil
- 2 pounds grass-fed cubed beef chuck roast

- Salt and freshly (finely ground) black pepper, as per taste preference

- 8-ounce chopped Portobello mushrooms

- 1 (15-ounce) can crushed tomatoes

- 1 (6-ounce) can tomato paste

- 1 seeded and chopped large green bell pepper

- 1 teaspoon crushed garlic

- 1 cup (preferably homemade) beef broth

Directions:

1. Season the meat with pepper and salt.

2. Arrange Instant Pot over a dry platform in your kitchen. Open its top lid and switch it on.

3. Find and press "SAUTE" cooking function; add the oil in it and allow it to heat.

4. In the pot, add the meat; cook (while stirring) until turns evenly brown from all sides for 4-5 minutes.

5. Stir in broth.

6. Close top lid to create a locked chamber; make sure that safety valve is in locking position.

7. Find and press "MANUAL" cooking function; timer to 15 minutes with default "HIGH" pressure mode.

8. Allow the pressure to build to cook the ingredients.

9. After cooking time is over, press "CANCEL" setting. Find and press "QPR" cooking function. This setting is for quick release of inside pressure.

10. Mix in the remaining ingredients.

11. Close top lid to create a locked chamber; make sure that safety valve is in locking position.

12. Find and press "MANUAL" cooking function; timer to 10 minutes with default "HIGH" pressure mode.

13. Allow the pressure to build to cook the ingredients.

14. After cooking time is over, press "CANCEL" setting. Find and press "NPR" cooking function. This setting is for natural release of inside pressure, and it takes around 10 minutes to slowly release pressure.

15. Slowly open the lid, take out the cooked recipe in serving plates or serving bowls and enjoy the keto recipe.

Nutritional Values (Per Serving):

Calories - 394

Fat – 32g

Saturated Fat – 6g

Trans Fat – 0g

Carbohydrates – 7g

Fiber – 3g

Sodium – 427mg

Protein – 33g

Turkey Tomato Meatballs

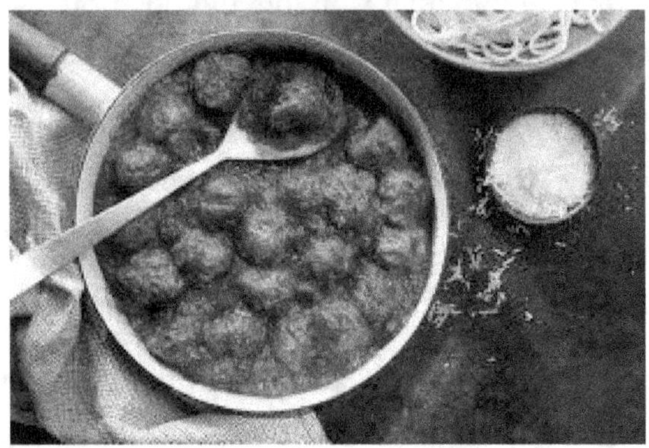

Prep Time: 8-10 min.

Cooking Time: 10 min.

Number of Servings: 4

Ingredients:

- 1/3 cup almond flour
- 3 ½ cups diced tomatoes
- 1 teaspoon basil
- 1 pound (finely ground) turkey
- 1/4 cup chicken stock
- 1/4 onion, diced
- 1 teaspoon minced garlic
- 1 teaspoon Italian seasoning
- (finely ground) black pepper and salt, as per taste preference

Directions:

1. Place the turkey, basil, onion, and almond flour in a bowl. Season with some (finely ground) black pepper and salt.

2. Make meatballs from the mixture.

3. Arrange Instant Pot over a dry platform in your kitchen. Open its top lid and switch it on.

4. Add the meatballs and other ingredients; gently stir to mix well.

5. Close top lid to create a locked chamber; make sure that safety valve is in locking position.

6. Find and press "MANUAL" cooking function; timer to 10 minutes with default "HIGH" pressure mode.

7. Allow the pressure to build to cook the ingredients.

8. After cooking time is over, press "CANCEL" setting. Find and press "QPR" cooking function. This setting is for quick release of inside pressure.

9. Slowly open the lid, take out the cooked recipe in serving plates or serving bowls and enjoy the keto recipe.

Nutritional Values (Per Serving):

Calories - 326

Fat – 14g

Saturated Fat – 2g

Trans Fat – 0g

Carbohydrates – 4g

Fiber – 1g

Sodium – 625mg

Protein – 27g

Chicken Zucchini Pasta

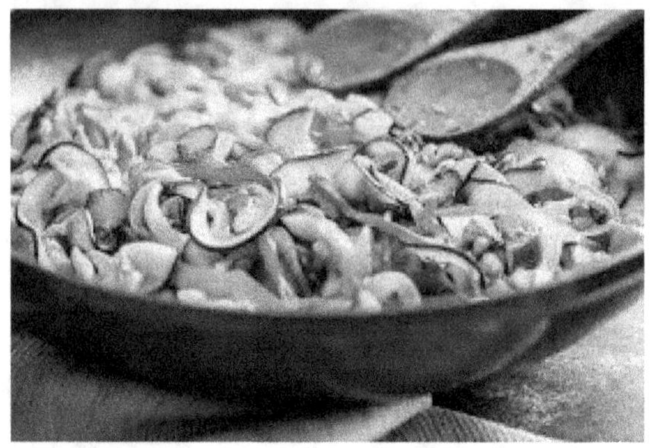

Prep Time: 8-10 min.

Cooking Time: 3 min.

Number of Servings: 3-4

Ingredients:

- 1 teaspoon Italian Seasoning
- 1 cup cooked and shredded Chicken
- 3 cups spiralized Zucchini
- 15 ounces low-carb Alfredo Sauce
- 3 tablespoons (grated or shredded) Parmesan Cheese
- (finely ground) black pepper and salt, as per taste preference

Directions:

1. Arrange Instant Pot over a dry platform in your kitchen. Open its top lid and switch it on.
2. Add the ingredients except for the cheese; season to taste and gently stir to mix well.

3. Close top lid to create a locked chamber; make sure that safety valve is in locking position.

4. Find and press "MANUAL" cooking function; timer to 3 minutes with default "HIGH" pressure mode.

5. Allow the pressure to build to cook the ingredients.

6. After cooking time is over, press "CANCEL" setting. Find and press "QPR" cooking function. This setting is for quick release of inside pressure.

7. Slowly open the lid, take out the cooked recipe in serving plates or serving bowls, top with the cheese and enjoy the keto recipe.

Nutritional Values (Per Serving):

Calories - 182

Fat – 11g

Saturated Fat – 3g

Trans Fat – 0g

Carbohydrates – 6g

Fiber – 1g

Sodium – 624mg

Protein – 14g

Super Herbed Fish

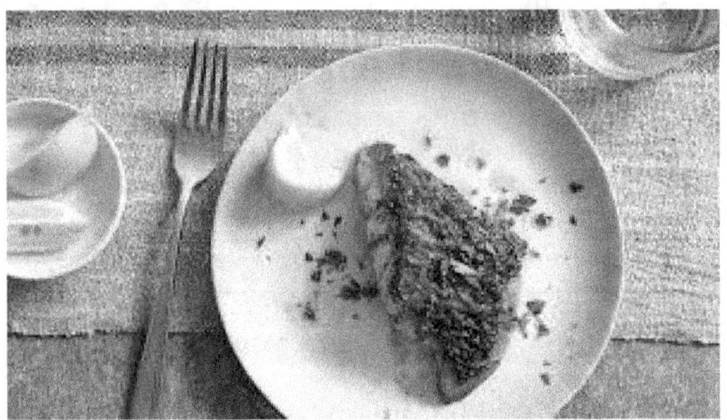

Prep Time: 8-10 min.

Cooking Time: 6 min.

Number of Servings: 1

Ingredients:

- 1 tablespoon chopped basil
- 2 teaspoons lime zest
- 1 tablespoon lime juice
- 1 tablespoon olive oil
- 1 4-ounce fish fillet
- 1 rosemary sprig
- 1 thyme sprig
- 1 teaspoon Dijon mustard
- ¼ teaspoon garlic powder
- Pinch of salt
- Pinch of pepper
- 1 ½ cups water

Directions:

1. Season the fish with salt and paper. Arrange on a piece of parchment paper and sprinkle with zest.

2. Whisk together the oil, juice, and mustard in a mixing bowl and brush over. Top with the herbs.

3. Wrap the fish with the parchment paper. Wrap the wrapped fish in an aluminum foil.

4. Arrange Instant Pot over a dry platform in your kitchen. Open its top lid and switch it on.

5. In the pot, pour water. Arrange a trivet or steamer basket inside that came with Instant Pot. Now place/arrange the foil over the trivet/basket.

6. Close top lid to create a locked chamber; make sure that safety valve is in locking position.

7. Find and press "MANUAL" cooking function; timer to 5 minutes with default "HIGH" pressure mode.

8. Allow the pressure to build to cook the ingredients.

9. After cooking time is over, press "CANCEL" setting. Find and press "QPR" cooking function. This setting is for quick release of inside pressure.

10. Slowly open the lid, take out the cooked recipe in serving plates or serving bowls and enjoy the keto recipe.

Nutritional Values (Per Serving):

Calories - 246

Fat – 9g

Saturated Fat – 1g

Trans Fat – 0g

Carbohydrates – 1g

Fiber – 0g

Sodium – 86mg

Protein – 28g

Turkey Avocado Chili

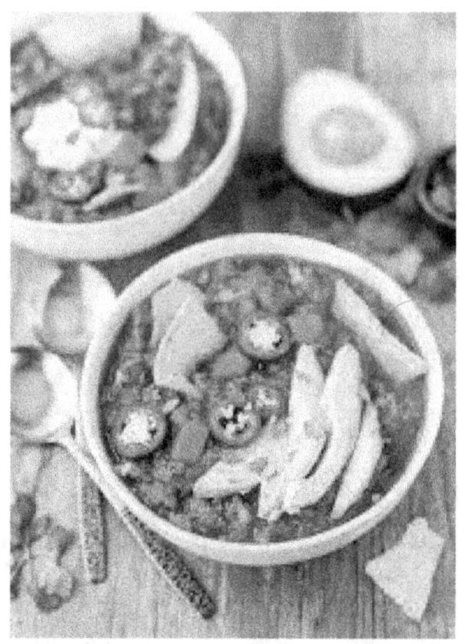

Prep Time: 8-10 min.

Cooking Time: 50 min.

Number of Servings: 3-4

Ingredients:

- 2 ½ pounds lean (finely ground) turkey

- 2 cups diced tomatoes

- 2-ounce tomato paste, sugar-free

- 1 tablespoon olive oil

- ½ chopped large yellow onion

- 8 minced garlic cloves

- 1 (4-ounce) can green chilies with liquid

- 2 tablespoons Worcestershire sauce

- 1 tablespoon dried oregano

- ¼ cup red chili powder

- 2 tablespoons (finely ground) cumin

- Salt and freshly (finely ground) black pepper, as per taste preference

- 1 pitted and sliced avocado, peeled

Directions:

1. Arrange Instant Pot over a dry platform in your kitchen. Open its top lid and switch it on.

2. Find and press "SAUTE" cooking function; add the oil in it and allow it to heat.

3. In the pot, add the onions; cook (while stirring) until turns translucent and softened for around 4-5 minutes.

4. Add the garlic and cook for about 1 minute.

5. Add the turkey and cook for about 8-9 minutes. Stir in remaining ingredients except for avocado.

6. Close top lid to create a locked chamber; make sure that safety valve is in locking position.

7. Find and press "MEAT/STEW" cooking function; timer to 35 minutes with default "HIGH" pressure mode.

8. Allow the pressure to build to cook the ingredients.

9. After cooking time is over, press "CANCEL" setting. Find and press "NPR" cooking function. This setting is for natural release of inside pressure and it takes around 10 minutes to slowly release pressure.

10. Slowly open the lid, take out the cooked recipe in serving plates or serving bowls, top with the avocado slices, and enjoy the keto recipe.

Nutritional Values (Per Serving):

Calories - 346

Fat – 19g

Saturated Fat – 4g

Trans Fat – 0g

Carbohydrates – 7g

Fiber – 5g

Sodium – 246mg

Protein – 29g

Cheesy Tomato Shrimp

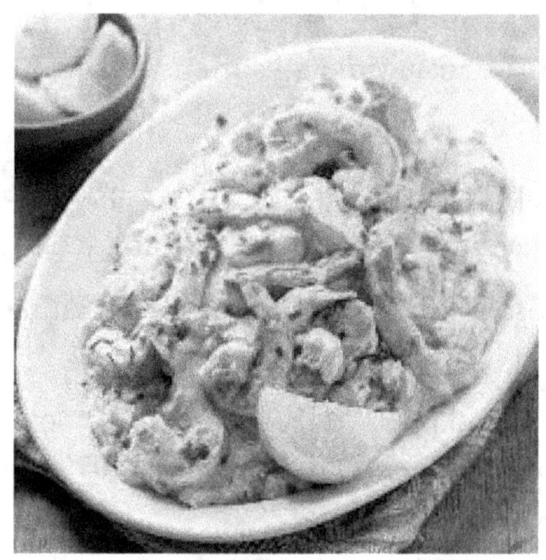

Prep Time: 8-10 min.

Cooking Time: 15 min.

Number of Servings: 4

Ingredients:

- 2 tablespoons olive oil
- ½ cup veggie broth
- ¼ cup chopped cilantro
- 2 tablespoons lime juice
- 1 ½ pounds shrimp, peeled and deveined
- 1 ½ pounds tomatoes, chopped
- 1 jalapeno, diced
- 1 onion, diced
- 1 cup shredded cheddar cheese
- 1 teaspoon minced garlic

Directions:

1. Arrange Instant Pot over a dry platform in your kitchen. Open its top lid and switch it on.

2. Find and press "SAUTE" cooking function; add the oil in it and allow it to heat.

3. In the pot, add the onions; cook (while stirring) until turns translucent and softened for around 2-3 minutes.

4. Add garlic and sauté for 30-60 seconds.

5. Stir in the broth, cilantro, and tomatoes.

6. Close top lid to create a locked chamber; make sure that safety valve is in locking position.

7. Find and press "MANUAL" cooking function; timer to 9 minutes with default "HIGH" pressure mode.

8. Allow the pressure to build to cook the ingredients.

9. After cooking time is over, press "CANCEL" setting. Find and press "NPR" cooking function. This setting is for natural release of inside pressure and it takes around 10 minutes to slowly release pressure.

10. Add the shrimps.

11. Close top lid to create a locked chamber; make sure that safety valve is in locking position.

12. Find and press "MANUAL" cooking function; timer to 2 minutes with default "HIGH" pressure mode.

13. Allow the pressure to build to cook the ingredients.

14. After cooking time is over, press "CANCEL" setting. Find and press "NPR" cooking function. This setting is for natural release of inside pressure, and it takes around 10 minutes to slowly release pressure.

15. Slowly open the lid, take out the cooked recipe in serving plates or serving bowls, top with the cheddar and enjoy the keto recipe.

Nutritional Values (Per Serving):

Calories - 268

Fat – 16g

Saturated Fat – 5g

Trans Fat – 0g

Carbohydrates – 8g

Fiber – 2g

Sodium – 208mg

Protein – 22g

Cajun Rosemary Chicken

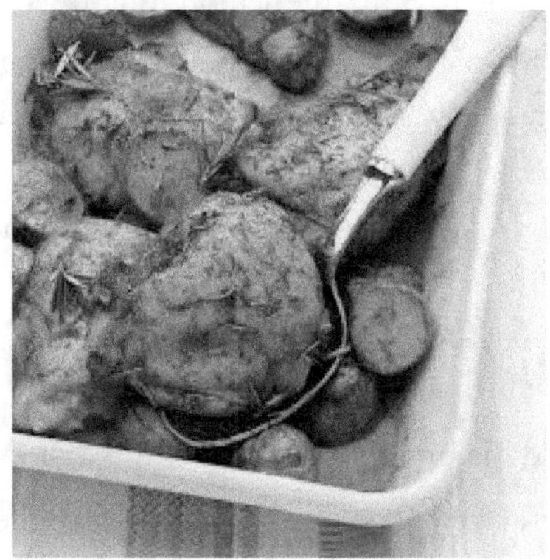

Prep Time: 8-10 min.

Cooking Time: 30 min.

Number of Servings: 4

Ingredients:

- 2 teaspoons Cajun seasoning
- 1 lemon, halved
- 1 yellow onion, make quarters
- 1 teaspoon garlic salt
- 1 medium chicken
- 2 rosemary sprigs
- 1 tablespoon coconut oil
- 1/4 teaspoon pepper
- 1 1/2 cups chicken broth

Directions:

1. Season the chicken with garlic salt, pepper, and Cajun seasoning. Stuff the lemon, onion, and rosemary in the chicken's cavity.

2. Arrange Instant Pot over a dry platform in your kitchen. Open its top lid and switch it on.

3. Find and press "SAUTE" cooking function; add the oil in it and allow it to heat.

4. In the pot, add the meat; cook (while stirring) until turns evenly brown from all sides.

5. Add the broth; gently stir to mix well.

6. Close top lid to create a locked chamber; make sure that safety valve is in locking position.

7. Find and press "MANUAL" cooking function; timer to 25 minutes with default "HIGH" pressure mode.

8. Allow the pressure to build to cook the ingredients.

9. After cooking time is over, press "CANCEL" setting. Find and press "NPR" cooking function. This setting is for natural release of inside pressure and it takes around 10 minutes to slowly release pressure.

10. Slowly open the lid, take out the cooked recipe in serving plates or serving bowls and enjoy the keto recipe.

Nutritional Values (Per Serving):

Calories - 236

Fat – 26g

Saturated Fat – 7g

Trans Fat – 0g

Carbohydrates – 1g

Fiber – 5g

Sodium – 426mg

Protein – 31g

Chicken Spinach Curry

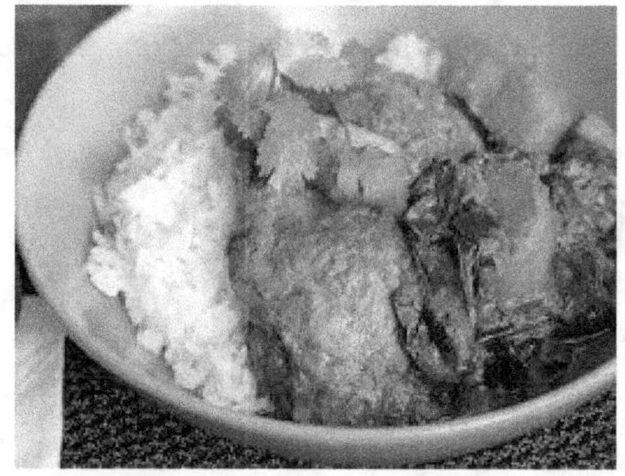

Prep Time: 8-10 min.

Cooking Time: 17 min.

Number of Servings: 3-4

Ingredients:

- 2 tomatoes, chopped
- 4 ounces spinach, chopped
- 1/3 pound curry paste
- 1 1/2 cups yogurt
- 4 pounds chicken, cubed
- 1 tablespoon olive oil
- 1 onion, cut to make slices
- 1 tablespoon chopped coriander

Directions:

1. Combine the chicken, curry paste, and yogurt in a mixing bowl. Cover and marinate in the fridge for 30 minutes.

2. Arrange Instant Pot over a dry platform in your kitchen. Open its top lid and switch it on.

3. Find and press "SAUTE" cooking function; add the oil in it and allow it to heat.

4. In the pot, add the onions; cook (while stirring) until turns translucent and softened.

5. Add the tomatoes and cook for another minute.

6. Pour the chicken mixture, mix in the spinach and coriander; gently stir to mix well.

7. Close top lid to create a locked chamber; make sure that safety valve is in locking position.

8. Find and press "MANUAL" cooking function; timer to 15 minutes with default "HIGH" pressure mode.

9. Allow the pressure to build to cook the ingredients.

10. After cooking time is over, press "CANCEL" setting. Find and press "QPR" cooking function. This setting is for quick release of inside pressure.

11. Slowly open the lid, take out the cooked recipe in serving plates or serving bowls and enjoy the keto recipe.

Nutritional Values (Per Serving):

Calories - 384

Fat – 18g

Saturated Fat – 3g

Trans Fat – 0g

Carbohydrates – 12g

Fiber – 6g

Sodium – 182mg
Protein – 39g

Chapter 8: Dinner

Pizza

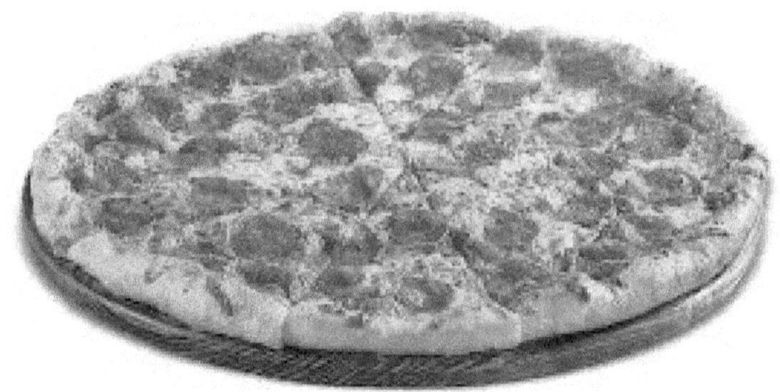

Prep time: 4 minutes

Cook time: 4 minutes

Number of Servings: 1

Ingredients

- 1 Tortilla Factory low carb whole wheat tortilla

- ¼ cup mozzarella cheese, hand-shredded

- ¼ cup tomato paste

- a sprinkle of Italian seasoning

- sprinkle with garlic salt

- Cut the broccoli, spinach, mushrooms, peppers, and onions you like for toppings

Directions

1. Turn broiler on in oven or toaster oven

2. Spread tortilla with tomato paste

3. Sprinkle seasoning on the paste

4. Add the cheese

5. Add the veggies

6. Broil or toast 1-4 minutes until crust is crunchy and cheese melted

7. Place when cooled into individual freezer bags. Microwave for 1 minute to refresh.

Nutritional Value:

Calories: 155,

Total Fat: 7g,

Protein: 13g,

Total Carbs: 18g,

Dietary Fiber: 10g,

Sugar: 2g,

Sodium: 741mg

Sriracha Tuna Kabobs

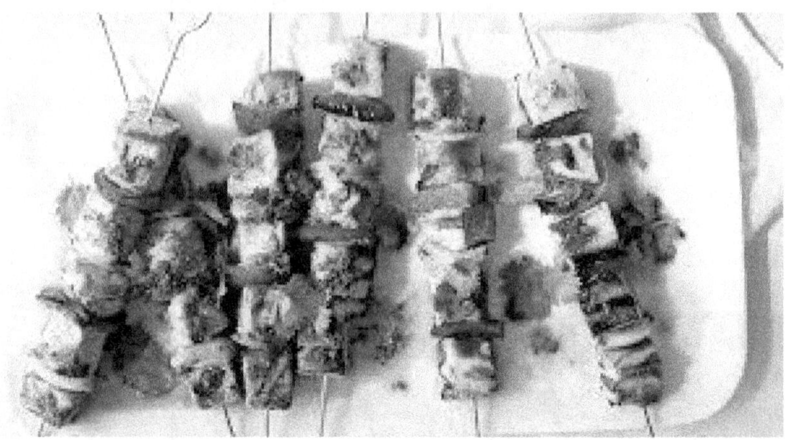

Prep time: 4 minutes

Cook time: 9 minutes

Number of Servings: 4

Ingredients

- 4 tablespoon Huy Fong chili garlic sauce

- 1 tablespoon sesame oil infused with garlic

- 1 tablespoon ginger, fresh, grated

- 1 tablespoon garlic, minced

- 1 red onion, cut into quarters and separated by petals

- 2 cups bell peppers, red, green, yellow

- 1 can whole water chestnuts, cut in half

- ½ pound fresh mushrooms, halved

- 32 oz. boneless tuna, chunks or steaks

- 1 Splenda packet

- 2 zucchini, sliced

- 1 inch thick, keep skins on

Directions

1. Layer the tuna and the vegetable pieces evenly onto 8 skewers.

2. Combine the spices and the oil and chili sauce, add the Splenda

3. Quickly blend, either in a blender or by Quickly whipping.

4. Brush onto the kabob pieces, make sure every piece is coated

5. Grill 4 minutes on each side, check to ensure the tuna is cooked to taste.

6. Serving size is two skewers.

7. Mix the marinade ingredients and store in covered container in the fridge. Place all the vegetables in one container in the fridge.

8. Place the tuna in a separate zip-lock bag.

Nutritional Value:

Calories: 467,

Total Fat: 18g,

Protein: 56g,

Total Carbs: 21g,

Dietary Fiber: 3.5g,

Sugar: 6g,

Sodium: 433mg

Chicken Relleno Casserole

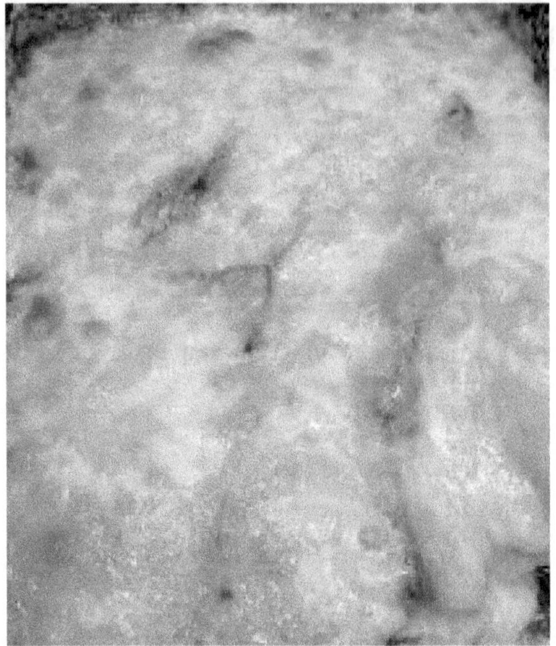

Prep time: 19 minutes

Cook time: 29 minutes

Number of Servings: 4

Ingredients

- 6 Tortilla Factory low-carb whole wheat tortillas, torn into small pieces

- 1 ½ cups hand-shredded cheese, Mexican

- 1 beaten egg

- 1 cup milk

- 2 cups cooked chicken, shredded

- 1 can Ro-tel

- ½ cup salsa verde

Directions

1. Grease an 8 x 8 glass baking dish

2. Heat oven to 375 degrees

3. Combine everything together, but reserve ½ cup of the cheese

4. Bake it for 29 minutes

5. Take it out of oven and add ½ cup cheese

6. Broil for about 2 minutes to melt the cheese

7. Let the casserole cool. Slice into 6 pieces and place in freezer containers, (1 cup with a lid) Freeze. Microwave for 2 minutes to serve. Top with sour cream, if desired.

Nutritional Value:

Calories: 265,

Total Fat: 16g,

Protein: 20g,

Total Carbs: 18g,

Dietary Fiber: 10g,

Sugar: 0g,

Sodium: 708mg

Steak Salad with Asian Spice

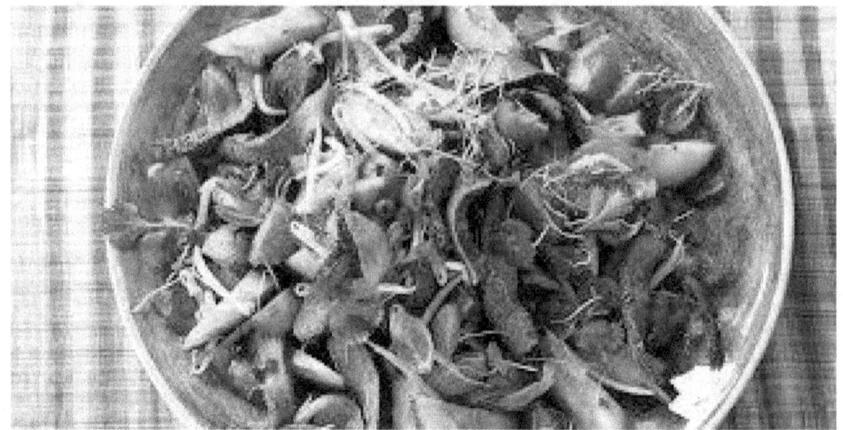

Prep time: 4 minutes

Cook time: 4 minutes

Number of Servings: 2

Ingredients

- 2 tablespoon sriracha sauce

- 1 tablespoon garlic, minced

- 1 tablespoon ginger, fresh, grated

- 1 bell pepper, yellow, cut into thin strips

- 1 bell pepper, red, cut into thin strips

- 1 tablespoon sesame oil, garlic

- 1 Splenda packet

- ½ tablespoon curry powder

- ½ tablespoon rice wine vinegar

- 8 oz. of beef sirloin, cut into strips

- 2 cups baby spinach, stemmed

- ½ head butter lettuce, torn or chopped into bite-sized pieces

Directions

1. Place the garlic, sriracha sauce, 1 tablespoon sesame oil, rice wine vinegar, and Splenda into a bowl and combine well.

2. Pour half of this mix into a zip-lock bag. Add the steak to marinade while you are preparing the salad.

3. Assemble the brightly colored salad by layering in two bowls.

4. Place the baby spinach into the bottom of the bowl. Place the butter lettuce next.

5. Mix the two peppers and place on top.

6. Remove the steak from the marinade and discard the liquid and bag.

7. Heat the sesame oil and quickly stir fry the steak until desired doneness, it should take about 3 minutes.

8. Place the steak on top of the salad.

9. Drizzle with the remaining dressing (other half of marinade mix).

10. Sprinkle sriracha sauce across the salad.

11. Combine the salad ingredients and place in a zip-lock bag in the fridge. Mix the marinade and halve into 2 zip-lock bags. Place the sriracha sauce into a small sealed container. Slice the steak and freeze in a zip-lock bag with the marinade. To prepare, mix the ingredients like the initial directions. Stir fry the marinated beef for 4 minutes to take into consideration the beef is frozen.

Nutritional Value:

Calories: 350,

Total Fat: 23g,

Protein: 28g,

Total Carbs: 7g,

Dietary Fiber: 3.5,

Sugar: 0,

Sodium: 267mg

Chicken Chow Mein Stir Fry

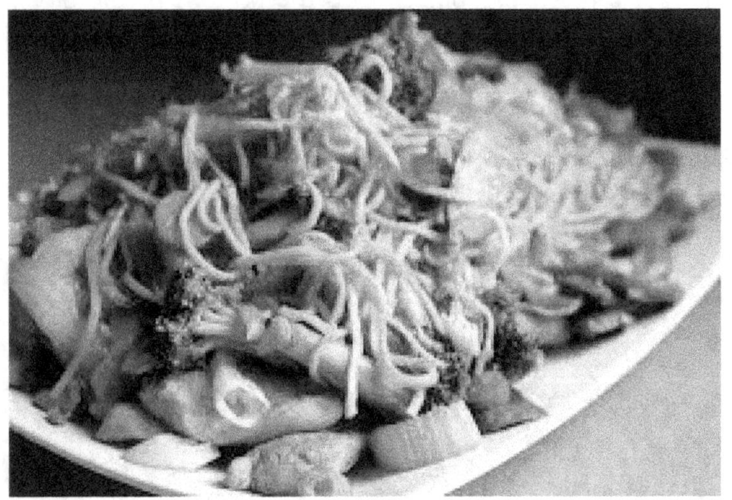

Prep time: 9 minutes

Cook time: 14 minutes

Number of Servings: 4

Ingredients

- 1/2 cup sliced onion

- 2 tablespoon Oil, sesame garlic flavored

- 4 cups shredded Bok-Choy

- 1 cup Sugar Snap Peas

- 1 cup fresh bean sprouts

- 3 stalks Celery, chopped

- 1 1/2 tablespoon minced Garlic

- 1 packet Splenda

- 1 cup Broth, chicken

- 2 tablespoon Soy Sauce

- 1 tablespoon ginger, freshly minced

- 1 tablespoon cornstarch

- 4 boneless Chicken Breasts, cooked/sliced thinly

Directions

1. Place the bok-choy, peas, celery in a skillet with 1 T garlic oil.

2. Stir fry until bok-choy is softened to liking.

3. Add remaining ingredients except for the cornstarch.

4. If too thin, stir cornstarch into ½ cup cold water. When smooth pour into skillet.

5. Bring cornstarch and chow mein to a one-minute boil. Turn off the heat source.

6. Stir sauce then for wait 4 minutes to serve, after the chow mein has thickened.

7. Freeze in covered containers. Heat for 2 minutes in the microwave before serving.

Nutritional Value:

Calories: 368,

Total Fat: 18g,

Protein: 42g,

Total Carbs: 12g,

Dietary Fiber: 16g,

Sugar: 6g,

Sodium: 746mg

Salmon with Bok-Choy

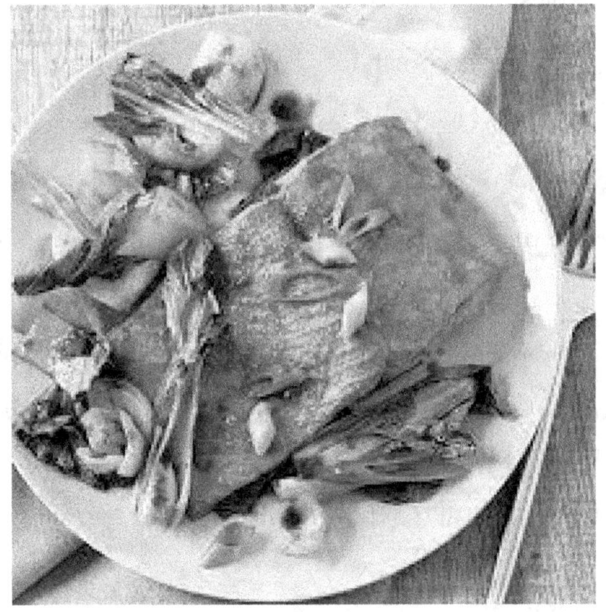

Prep time: 9 minutes

Cook time: 9 minutes

Number of Servings: 4

Ingredients

- 1 cup red peppers, roasted, drained

- 2 cups chopped bok-choy

- 1 tablespoon salted butter

- 5 oz. salmon steak

- 1 lemon, sliced very thinly

- ⅛ tablespoon black pepper

- 1 tablespoon olive oil

- 2 tablespoon sriracha sauce

Directions

1. Place oil in skillet

2. Place all but 4 slices of lemon in the skillet.

3. Sprinkle the bok choy with the black pepper.

4. Stir fry the bok-choy with the lemons.

5. Remove and place on four plates.

6. Place the butter in the skillet and stir fry the salmon, turning once.

7. Place the salmon on the bed of bok-choy.

8. Divide the red peppers and encircle the salmon.

9. Place a slice of lemon atop the salmon.

10. Drizzle with sriracha sauce.

11. Freeze the cooked salmon in individual zip-lock bags. Place the bok-choy, with the remaining ingredients into one cup containers. Microwave the salmon for one minute and the frozen bok choy for two. Assemble to serve.

Nutritional Value:

Calories: 410,

Total Fat: 30g,

Protein: 30g,

Total Carbs: 7g,

Dietary Fiber: 2g,

Sugar: 0g,

Sodium: 200mg

Chapter 9: Soups & Stews

Mushroom Pork Stew

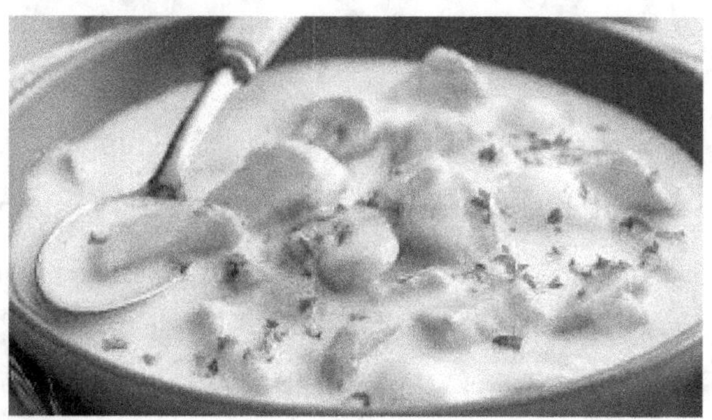

Prep Time: 8-10 min.

Cooking Time: 60 min.

Number of Servings: 3-4

Ingredients:

- 4 pounds pork cheeks
- 2 cups white mushrooms, cut to make slices
- 1 1/2 cups water
- 4 tablespoons avocado or coconut oil
- 6 cloves of garlic, minced
- 1 onion diced
- Juice from 1 lemon
- (finely ground) black pepper and salt as per taste preference

Directions:

1. Arrange Instant Pot over a dry platform in your kitchen. Open its top lid and switch it on.

2. Find and press "SAUTE" cooking function; add the oil in it and allow it to heat.

3. In the pot, add the onions, garlic; cook (while stirring) until turns translucent and softened for around 1-2 minutes.

4. Stir in the pork cheeks; cook for 2 minutes.

5. Add the remaining ingredients; gently stir to mix well.

6. Close top lid to create a locked chamber; make sure that safety valve is in locking position.

7. Find and press "MEAT/STEW" cooking function; timer to 55 minutes with default "HIGH" pressure mode.

8. Allow the pressure to build to cook the ingredients.

9. After cooking time is over, press "CANCEL" setting. Find and press "QPR" cooking function. This setting is for quick release of inside pressure.

10. Slowly open the lid, take out the cooked recipe in serving plates or serving bowls and enjoy the keto recipe.

Nutritional Values (Per Serving):

Calories - 361

Fat – 32g

Saturated Fat – 8g

Trans Fat – 0g

Carbohydrates – 4g

Fiber – 1g

Sodium – 172mg

Protein – 26g

Broccoli Chicken Stew

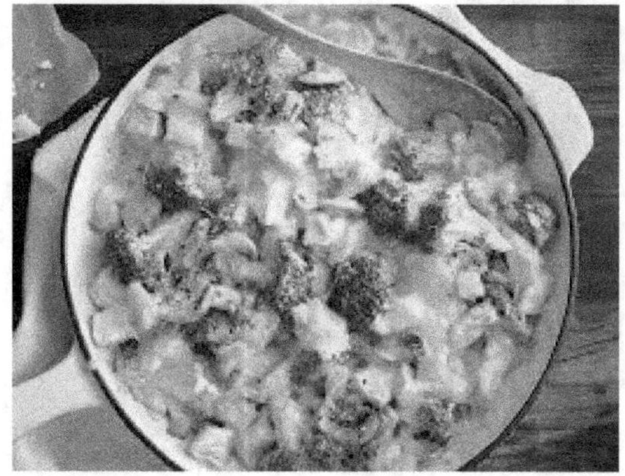

Prep Time: 8-10 min.

Cooking Time: 10 min.

Number of Servings: 4

Ingredients:

- 1 cup chopped cauliflower
- 1 onion, finely chopped
- 1 tomato, chopped
- 1 whole chicken
- 10 ounce broccoli
- 3 tablespoon olive oil
- 4 cups chicken broth
- 2 teaspoon salt
- 1 tablespoon cayenne pepper
- ½ teaspoon black pepper

Directions:

1. Season the chicken with salt. Set aside.

2. Arrange Instant Pot over a dry platform in your kitchen. Open its top lid and switch it on.

3. Find and press "SAUTE" cooking function; add the oil in it and allow it to heat.

4. In the pot, add the onions; cook (while stirring) until turns translucent and softened for around 3-4 minutes.

5. Add the tomato; cook for another 5 minutes, stirring constantly.

6. Add the other ingredients; gently stir to mix well.

7. Close top lid to create a locked chamber; make sure that safety valve is in locking position.

8. Find and press "MANUAL" cooking function; timer to 30 minutes with default "HIGH" pressure mode.

9. Allow the pressure to build to cook the ingredients.

10. After cooking time is over, press "CANCEL" setting. Find and press "NPR" cooking function. This setting is for natural release of inside pressure and it takes around 10 minutes to slowly release pressure.

11. Slowly open the lid, take out the cooked recipe in serving plates or serving bowls and enjoy the keto recipe.

Nutritional Values (Per Serving):

Calories - 523

Fat – 17g

Saturated Fat – 4g

Trans Fat – 0g

Carbohydrates – 9g

Fiber – 3g

Sodium – 628mg

Cream Zucchini Soup

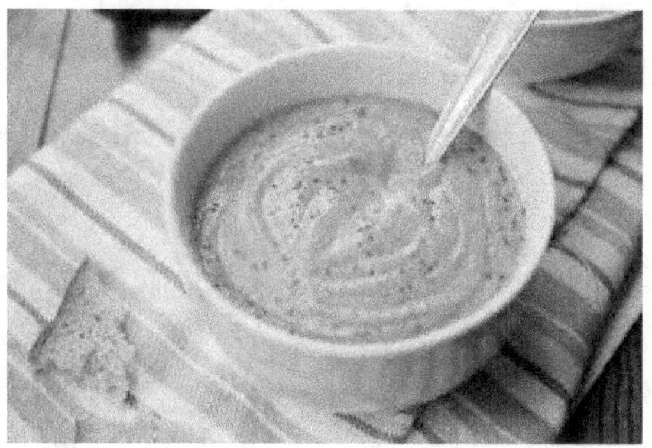

Prep Time: 8-10 min.

Cooking Time: 8 min.

Number of Servings: 4

Ingredients:

- 2 cups vegetable stock
- 2 garlic cloves, crushed
- 1 tablespoon butter
- 4 (preferably medium size) zucchinis, peeled and chopped
- 1 small onion, chopped
- 2 cups heavy cream
- 1/2 teaspoon dried oregano, (finely ground)
- 1/2 teaspoon black pepper, (finely ground)
- 1 teaspoon dried parsley, (finely ground)
- 1 teaspoon sea salt

- Lemon juice (optional)

Directions:

1. Arrange Instant Pot over a dry platform in your kitchen. Open its top lid and switch it on.

2. Find and press "SAUTE" cooking function; add the butter in it and allow it to melt.

3. In the pot, add the onions, zucchini, garlic; cook (while stirring) until turns translucent and softened for around 2-3 minutes.

4. Add the vegetable broth and sprinkle with salt, oregano, pepper, and parsley; gently stir to mix well.

5. Close top lid to create a locked chamber; make sure that safety valve is in locking position.

6. Find and press "MANUAL" cooking function; timer to 5 minutes with default "HIGH" pressure mode.

7. Allow the pressure to build to cook the ingredients.

8. After cooking time is over, press "CANCEL" setting. Find and press "QPR" cooking function. This setting is for quick release of inside pressure.

9. Slowly open the lid, take out the cooked recipe in serving plates or serving bowls and enjoy the keto recipe. Top with some lemon juice.

Nutritional Values (Per Serving):

Calories - 264

Fat – 26g

Saturated Fat – 7g

Trans Fat – 0g

Carbohydrates – 11g

Fiber – 3g

Sodium – 564mg

Protein – 4g

Coconut Chicken Soup

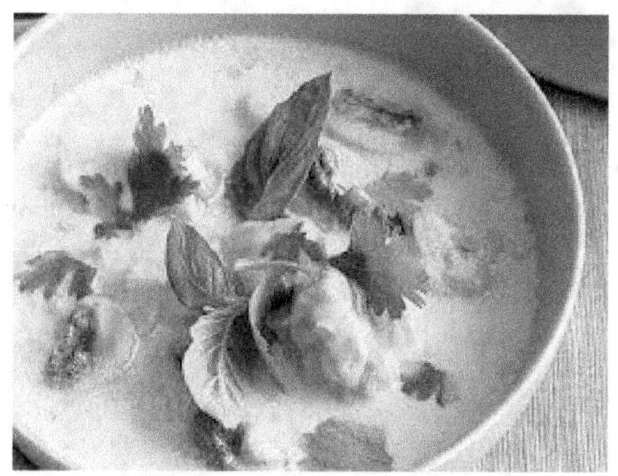

Prep Time: 8-10 min.

Cooking Time: 18 min.

Number of Servings: 4

Ingredients:

- 4 cloves of garlic, minced
- 1 pound chicken breasts, skin-on
- 4 cups water
- 2 tablespoons olive oil
- 1 onion, diced
- 1 cup coconut milk
- (finely ground) black pepper and salt as per taste preference
- 2 tablespoons sesame oil

Directions:

1. Arrange Instant Pot over a dry platform in your kitchen. Open its top lid and switch it on.

2. Find and press "SAUTE" cooking function; add the oil in it and allow it to heat.

3. In the pot, add the onions, garlic; cook (while stirring) until turns translucent and softened for around 1-2 minutes.

4. Stir in the chicken breasts; stir-cook for 2 more minutes.

5. Pour in water and coconut milk. Season to taste.

6. Close top lid to create a locked chamber; make sure that safety valve is in locking position.

7. Find and press "MANUAL" cooking function; timer to 15 minutes with default "HIGH" pressure mode.

8. Allow the pressure to build to cook the ingredients.

9. After cooking time is over, press "CANCEL" setting. Find and press "NPR" cooking function. This setting is for natural release of inside pressure and it takes around 10 minutes to slowly release pressure.

10. Slowly open the lid, Drizzle with sesame oil on top.

11. Take out the cooked recipe in serving plates or serving bowls and enjoy the keto recipe.

Nutritional Values (Per Serving):

Calories - 328

Fat – 31g

Saturated Fat – 6g

Trans Fat – 0g

Carbohydrates – 6g

Fiber – 4g

Sodium – 76mg

Protein – 21g

Chicken Bacon Soup

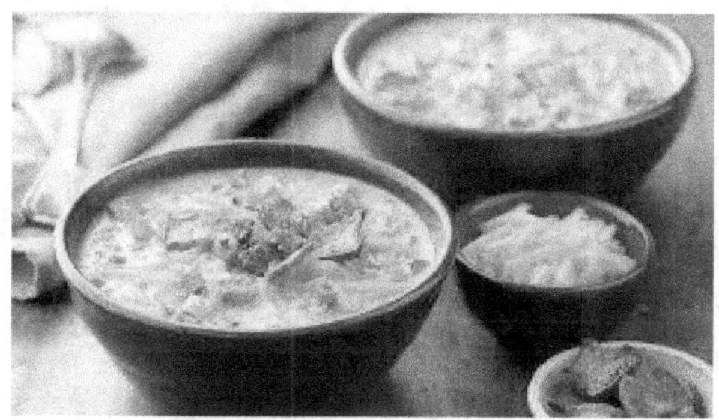

Prep Time: 8-10 min.

Cooking Time: 40 min.

Number of Servings: 4

Ingredients:

- 6 boneless, skinless chicken thighs, make cubes
- ½ cup chopped celery
- 4 minced garlic cloves
- 6-ounce mushrooms, sliced
- ½ cup chopped onion
- 8-ounce softened cream cheese
- ¼ cup softened butter
- 1 teaspoon dried thyme
- Salt and (finely ground) black pepper, as per taste preference

- 2 cups chopped spinach

- 8 ounces cooked bacon slices, chopped

- 3 cups (preferably homemade) chicken broth

- 1 cup heavy cream

Directions:

1. Arrange Instant Pot over a dry platform in your kitchen. Open its top lid and switch it on.

2. Add the ingredients except for the cream, spinach and bacon; gently stir to mix well.

3. Close top lid to create a locked chamber; make sure that safety valve is in locking position.

4. Find and press "SOUP" cooking function; timer to 30 minutes with default "HIGH" pressure mode.

5. Allow the pressure to build to cook the ingredients.

6. After cooking time is over, press "CANCEL" setting. Find and press "NPR" cooking function. This setting is for natural release of inside pressure and it takes around 10 minutes to slowly release pressure.

7. Slowly open the lid, stir in cream and spinach.

8. take out the cooked recipe in serving plates or serving bowls and enjoy the keto recipe. Top with the bacon.

Nutritional Values (Per Serving):

Calories - 456

Fat – 38g

Saturated Fat – 13g

Trans Fat – 0g

Carbohydrates – 6g

Fiber – 1g

Sodium – 742mg

Protein – 23g

Cream Pepper Stew

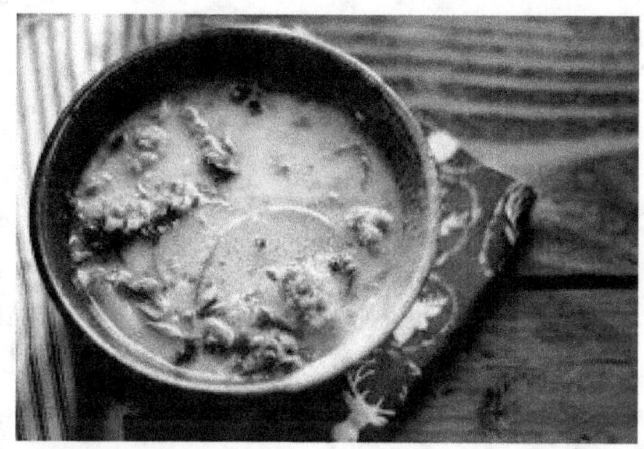

Prep Time: 8-10 min.

Cooking Time: 10 min.

Number of Servings: 4

Ingredients:

- 1 (preferably medium size) celery stalk, chopped
- 1 (preferably medium size) yellow bell pepper, chopped
- 1 (preferably medium size) green bell pepper, chopped
- 2 large red bell peppers, chopped
- 1 small red onion, chopped
- 2 tablespoons butter
- 1/2 cup cream cheese, full-fat
- 1/4 teaspoon dried thyme, (finely ground)
- 1/2 teaspoon black pepper, (finely ground)

- 1 teaspoon dried parsley, (finely ground)

- 1 teaspoon salt

- 2 cups vegetable stock

- 1 cup heavy cream

Directions:

1. Arrange Instant Pot over a dry platform in your kitchen. Open its top lid and switch it on.

2. Find and press "SAUTE" cooking function; add the butter in it and allow it to heat.

3. In the pot, add the onions, bell pepper, and celery; cook (while stirring) until turns translucent and softened for around 3-4 minutes.

4. Pour in the vegetable stock and heavy cream. Season with salt, pepper, parsley, and thyme.

5. Close top lid to create a locked chamber; make sure that safety valve is in locking position.

6. Find and press "MANUAL" cooking function; timer to 6 minutes with default "HIGH" pressure mode.

7. Allow the pressure to build to cook the ingredients.

8. After cooking time is over, press "CANCEL" setting. Find and press "QPR" cooking function. This setting is for quick release of inside pressure.

9. Slowly open the lid, mix in the cream; take out the cooked recipe in serving plates or serving bowls and enjoy the keto recipe.

Nutritional Values (Per Serving):

Calories - 286

Fat – 27g

Saturated Fat – 6g

Trans Fat – 0g

Carbohydrates – 9g

Fiber – 3g

Sodium – 523mg

Protein – 5g

Ham Asparagus Soup

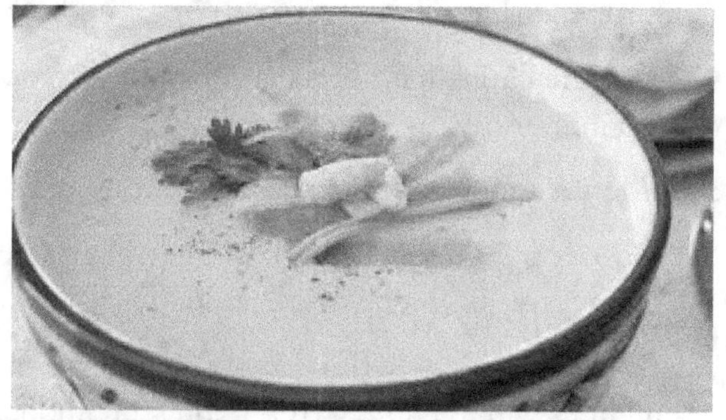

Prep Time: 8-10 min.

Cooking Time: 55 min.

Number of Servings: 3-4

Ingredients:

- 5 crushed garlic cloves
- 1 cup chopped ham
- 4 cups (preferably homemade) chicken broth
- 2 pounds trimmed and halved asparagus spears
- 2 tablespoons butter
- 1 chopped yellow onion
- ½ teaspoon dried thyme

- Salt and freshly (finely ground) black pepper, as per taste preference

Directions:

1. Arrange Instant Pot over a dry platform in your kitchen. Open its top lid and switch it on.

2. Find and press "SAUTE" cooking function; add the butter in it and allow it to heat.

3. In the pot, add the onions; cook (while stirring) until turns translucent and softened for around 4-5 minutes.

4. Add the garlic, ham bone and broth; stir-cook for about 2-3 minutes.

5. Add the other ingredients; gently stir to mix well.

6. Close top lid to create a locked chamber; make sure that safety valve is in locking position.

7. Find and press "SOUP" cooking function; timer to 45 minutes with default "HIGH" pressure mode.

8. Allow the pressure to build to cook the ingredients.

9. After cooking time is over, press "CANCEL" setting. Find and press "QPR" cooking function. This setting is for quick release of inside pressure.

10. Slowly open the lid, add the prepared recipe mix in a blender or processor.

11. Blend or process to make a smooth mix. Place the mix in serving bowls and enjoy the keto recipe.

Nutritional Values (Per Serving):

Calories - 146

Fat – 7g

Saturated Fat – 3g

Trans Fat – 0g

Carbohydrates – 5g

Fiber – 4g

Sodium – 262mg

Protein – 10g

Chapter 10: Delicious Desserts

Almond Mug Cake

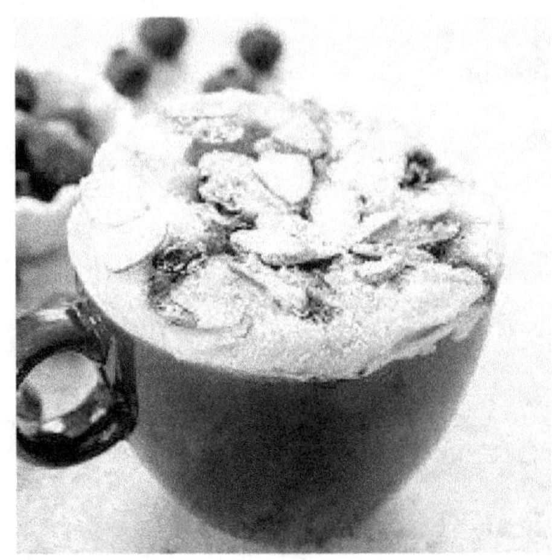

Prep Time: 8-10 min.

Cooking Time: 10 min.

Number of Servings: 1

Ingredients:

- 1/4 teaspoon baking powder
- 1/4 teaspoon vanilla extract
- 1 1/2 tablespoons cacao powder
- 1 egg, beaten
- 1/4 cup almond flour
- 1 teaspoon cinnamon powder
- 2 tablespoons stevia powder
- A pinch of salt

Directions:

1. Combine all ingredients in the bowl until well-combined. Add the mix in a heat-proof mug; cover with a foil.

2. Arrange Instant Pot over a dry platform in your kitchen. Open its top lid and switch it on.

3. In the pot, pour water. Arrange a trivet or steamer basket inside that came with Instant Pot. Now place/arrange the mug over the trivet/basket.

4. Close top lid to create a locked chamber; make sure that safety valve is in locking position.

5. Find and press "MANUAL" cooking function; timer to 10 minutes with default "HIGH" pressure mode.

6. Allow the pressure to build to cook the ingredients.

7. After cooking time is over, press "CANCEL" setting. Find and press "QPR" cooking function. This setting is for quick release of inside pressure.

8. Slowly open the lid, cool down the mug and serve warm.

Nutritional Values (Per Serving):

Calories - 138

Fat – 13g

Saturated Fat – 6g

Trans Fat – 0g

Carbohydrates – 7g

Fiber – 3g

Sodium – 73mg

Protein – 9g

Tapioca Keto Pudding

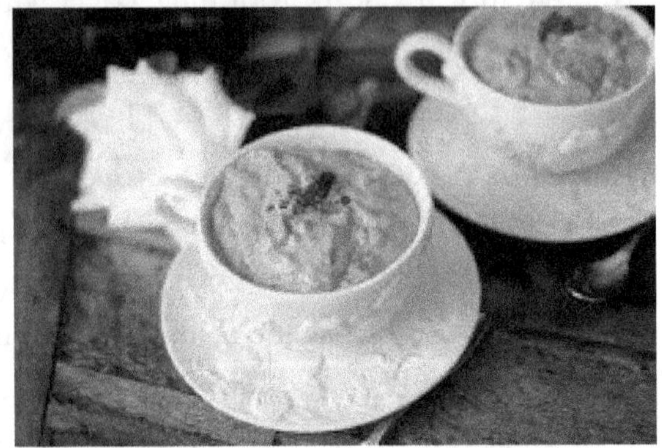

Prep Time: 8-10 min.

Cooking Time: 20 min.

Number of Servings: 4

Ingredients:

- 1 tablespoon Erythritol
- 1 teaspoon chia seeds
- 1 tablespoon tapioca
- 1 tablespoon butter
- 2 cup heavy cream
- 1/4 cup raspberries or strawberries, mashed

Directions:

1. Arrange Instant Pot over a dry platform in your kitchen. Open its top lid and switch it on.

2. Find and press "SAUTE" cooking function.

3. In the pot, add the cream; cook (while stirring) for 4-5 minutes.

4. Add the tapioca and stir it well. Add the Erythritol and butter.

5. In a bowl, mix the chia seeds and berries.

6. Add the berry mix in the pot and stir well.

7. Close top lid to create a locked chamber; make sure that safety valve is in locking position.

8. Find and press "MANUAL" cooking function; timer to 15 minutes with default "HIGH" pressure mode.

9. Allow the pressure to build to cook the ingredients.

10. After cooking time is over, press "CANCEL" setting. Find and press "QPR" cooking function. This setting is for quick release of inside pressure.

11. Add in serving bowls, cool down and place in the fridge for 2 hours.

12. Serve chilled.

Nutritional Values (Per Serving):

Calories - 246

Fat – 24g

Saturated Fat – 9g

Trans Fat – 0g

Carbohydrates – 10g

Fiber – 2g

Sodium – 183mg

Protein – 3g

Cream Chocolate Delight

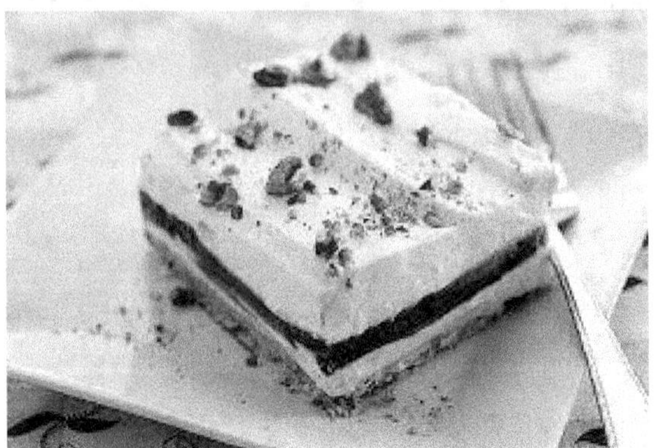

Prep Time: 8-10 min.

Cooking Time: 15 min.

Number of Servings: 4

Ingredients:

- 1 teaspoon orange zest
- 1 teaspoon stevia powder
- 2 heavy cream
- ¼ cup unsweetened dark chocolate, chopped
- 3 eggs
- 1 teaspoon vanilla extract
- ½ teaspoon salt

Directions:

1. Arrange Instant Pot over a dry platform in your kitchen. Open its top lid and switch it on.

2. Find and press "SAUTE" cooking function.

3. In the pot, add the heavy cream, chopped chocolate, stevia powder, vanilla extract, orange zest, and salt; cook (while stirring) until the chocolate is melted.

4. Crack eggs in the pot; stirring constantly. Remove from the instant pot. Add the mixture to 4 mason jars with loose lids.

5. In the pot, pour water. Arrange a trivet or steamer basket inside that came with Instant Pot. Now place/arrange the jars over the trivet/basket.

6. Close top lid to create a locked chamber; make sure that safety valve is in locking position.

7. Find and press "MANUAL" cooking function; timer to 10 minutes with default "HIGH" pressure mode.

8. Allow the pressure to build to cook the ingredients.

9. After cooking time is over, press "CANCEL" setting. Find and press "QPR" cooking function. This setting is for quick release of inside pressure.

10. Slowly open the lid, cool down the jars and chill in the fridge. Serve chilled.

Nutritional Values (Per Serving):

Calories - 254

Fat – 26g

Saturated Fat – 12g

Trans Fat – 0g

Carbohydrates – 5g

Fiber – 1g

Sodium – 168mg

Protein – 8g

Coconut Keto Pudding

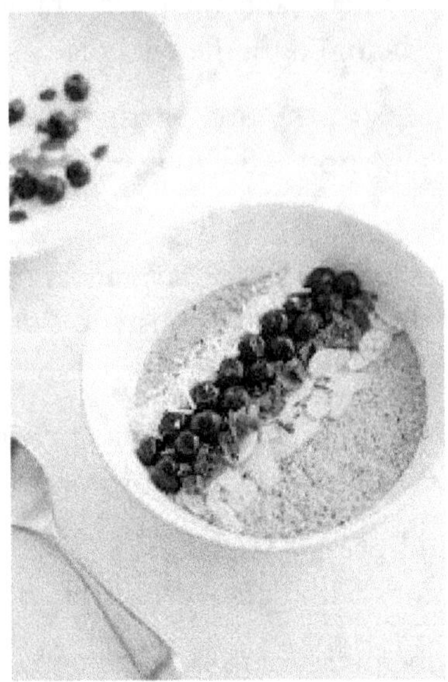

Prep Time: 8-10 min.

Cooking Time: 5 min.

Number of Servings: 4

Ingredients:

- 3 tablespoons Stevia granular
- 1/2 teaspoon vanilla extract
- 1 2/3 cup coconut milk
- 3 egg yolks
- 1 tablespoon gelatin

Directions:

1. Arrange Instant Pot over a dry platform in your kitchen. Open its top lid and switch it on.
2. Add the coconut milk.

3. Close top lid to create a locked chamber; make sure that safety valve is in locking position.

4. Find and press "MANUAL" cooking function; timer to 5 minutes with default "HIGH" pressure mode.

5. Allow the pressure to build to cook the ingredients.

6. After cooking time is over, press "CANCEL" setting. Find and press "QPR" cooking function. This setting is for quick release of inside pressure.

7. Place the coconut milk in the Instant Pot. Close the lid and make sure that the steam release valve is set to "Sealing."

8. Whisk in egg yolks and the rest of the ingredients.

9. Find and press "SAUTE" cooking function. Cook until boiling the mix.

10. Add in serving bowls, cool down and place in the fridge for 2 hours.

11. Serve chilled.

Nutritional Values (Per Serving):

Calories - 246

Fat – 27g

Saturated Fat – 8g

Trans Fat – 0g

Carbohydrates – 7g

Fiber – 4g

Sodium – 89mg

Protein – 4g

Vanilla Cream Delight

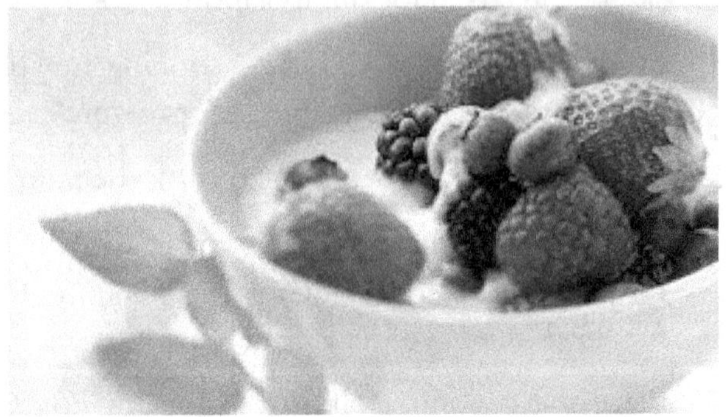

Prep Time: 8-10 min.

Cooking Time: 15 min.

Number of Servings: 4

Ingredients:

- 1 ½ cup heavy cream
- 1 teaspoon vanilla extract
- 8 large eggs
- ¾ cup unsweetened almond milk
- 1 vanilla bean
- 4 tablespoons stevia granular

Directions:

1. Cut the vanilla bean lengthwise using a knife and take out the seeds. Add in a mixing bowl.

2. Mix in the remaining ingredients. Whisk the mix thoroughly and add into 4 ramekins.

3. Arrange Instant Pot over a dry platform in your kitchen. Open its top lid and switch it on.

4. In the pot, pour 2 cups water. Arrange a trivet or steamer basket inside that came with Instant Pot. Now place/arrange the ramekins over the trivet/basket.

5. Close top lid to create a locked chamber; make sure that safety valve is in locking position.

6. Find and press "MANUAL" cooking function; timer to 15 minutes with default "HIGH" pressure mode.

7. Allow the pressure to build to cook the ingredients.

8. After cooking time is over, press "CANCEL" setting. Find and press "QPR" cooking function. This setting is for quick release of inside pressure.

9. Slowly open the lid, cool down the ramekins.

10. Chill in fridge and serve.

Nutritional Values (Per Serving):

Calories - 318

Fat – 26g

Saturated Fat – 7g

Trans Fat – 0g

Carbohydrates – 3g

Fiber – 0g

Sodium – 106mg

Protein – 13g

Chapter 11: Snacks & Dips

Spinach Mayo Dip

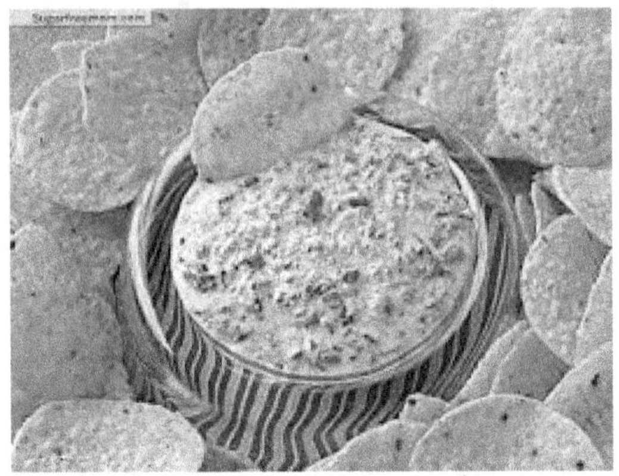

Prep Time: 8-10 min.

Cooking Time: 7 min.

Number of Servings: 4

Ingredients:

- ½ cup (preferably homemade) chicken broth
- 8-ounce cubed cream cheese
- 1 cup shredded mozzarella cheese
- 1 tablespoon olive oil
- 1 pound spinach, chopped
- 3 minced garlic cloves
- ½ cup mayonnaise
- ½ cup sour cream
- 1 teaspoon onion powder
- Salt and (finely ground) black pepper, as per taste preference

Directions:

1. Arrange Instant Pot over a dry platform in your kitchen. Open its top lid and switch it on.

2. Find and press "SAUTE" cooking function; add the oil in it and allow it to heat.

3. In the pot, add the garlic, spinach; cook (while stirring) until turns translucent and softened for around 2-3 minutes.

4. Add the remaining ingredients and stir to combine.

5. Close top lid to create a locked chamber; make sure that safety valve is in locking position.

6. Find and press "MANUAL" cooking function; timer to 4 minutes with default "HIGH" pressure mode.

7. Allow the pressure to build to cook the ingredients.

8. After cooking time is over, press "CANCEL" setting. Find and press "QPR" cooking function. This setting is for quick release of inside pressure.

9. Slowly open the lid, take out the cooked recipe in serving plates or serving bowls and enjoy the keto recipe.

Nutritional Values (Per Serving):

Calories – 246

Fat – 20g

Saturated Fat – 6g

Trans Fat – 0g

Carbohydrates – 4g

Fiber – 0.3g

Sodium – 423mg

Protein – 5g

Parmesan Asparagus

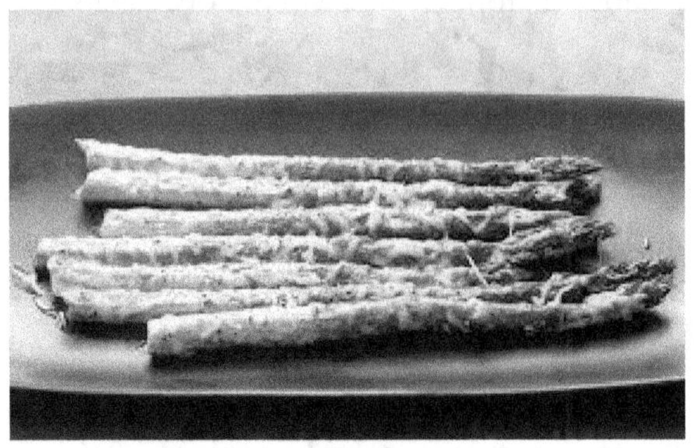

Prep Time: 10 min.

Cooking Time: 8 min.

Number of Servings: 4

Ingredients:

- 3 tablespoons full-fat butter

- 3 tablespoons (grated or shredded) Parmesan cheese

- 1 pound trimmed asparagus

- 3 garlic cloves

Directions:

1. Arrange the asparagus and garlic in a large piece of foil and top with butter.

2. Fold the edges to make a pocket.

1. Arrange Instant Pot over a dry platform in your kitchen. Open its top lid and switch it on.

2. In the pot, pour 1 cup water. Arrange a trivet or steamer basket inside that came with Instant Pot. Now place/arrange the pocket over the trivet/basket.

3. Close top lid to create a locked chamber; make sure that safety valve is in locking position.

4. Find and press "STEAM" cooking function; timer to 8 minutes with default "HIGH" pressure mode.

5. Allow the pressure to build to cook the ingredients.

6. After cooking time is over, press "CANCEL" setting. Find and press "QPR" cooking function. This setting is for quick release of inside pressure.

7. Slowly open the lid, take out the cooked recipe in serving plates or serving bowls, top with the cheese and enjoy the keto recipe.

Nutritional Values (Per Serving):

Calories - 114

Fat – 10g

Saturated Fat – 3g

Trans Fat – 0g

Carbohydrates – 3g

Fiber – 2g

Sodium – 86mg

Protein – 3g

Cauliflower Yogurt Mash Dip

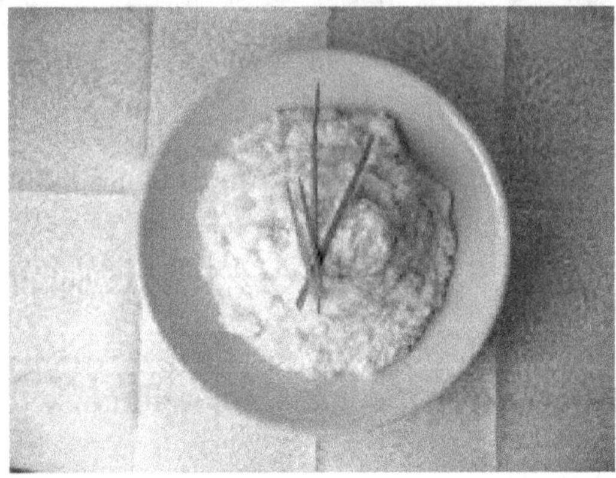

Prep Time: 10-15 min.

Cooking Time: 3 min.

Number of Servings: 3-4

Ingredients:

- 2 tablespoons plain Greek yogurt

- Salt and (finely ground) black pepper, as per taste preference

- 2 teaspoons melted butter

- ½ cup (preferably homemade) chicken broth

- 1 chopped head cauliflower

- 2 tablespoons chopped chives

Directions:

1. Arrange Instant Pot over a dry platform in your kitchen. Open its top lid and switch it on.

2. In the pot, pour broth. Arrange a trivet or steamer basket inside that came with Instant Pot. Now place/arrange the cauliflower over the trivet/basket.

3. Close top lid to create a locked chamber; make sure that safety valve is in locking position.

4. Find and press "MANUAL" cooking function; timer to 3 minutes with default "HIGH" pressure mode.

5. Allow the pressure to build to cook the ingredients.

6. After cooking time is over, press "CANCEL" setting. Find and press "QPR" cooking function. This setting is for quick release of inside pressure.

7. Add the cauliflower into a food processor or blender.

8. Add yogurt, salt, and black pepper; blend until smooth.

9. Add the mashed cauliflower to a serving bowl. Drizzle with the ghee and chives.

Nutritional Values (Per Serving):

Calories - 38

Fat – 4g

Saturated Fat – 1g

Trans Fat – 0g

Carbohydrates – 3g

Fiber – 2g

Sodium – 76mg

Protein – 3g

Avocado Keto Eggs

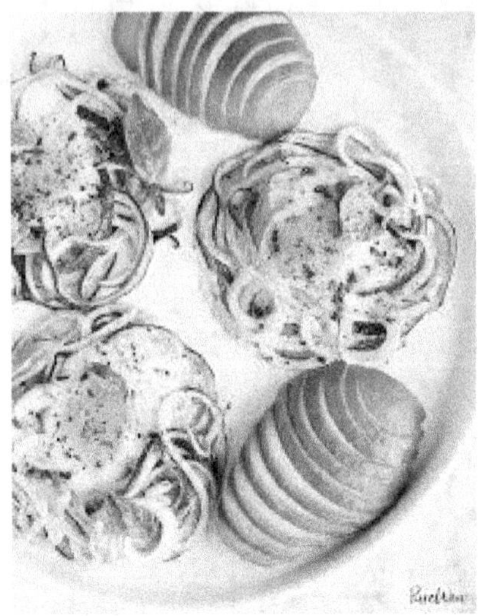

Prep Time: 8-10 min.

Cooking Time: 6 min.

Number of Servings: 4

Ingredients:

- 6 large eggs
- 1 minced serrano chili, minced
- 1 tablespoon lime juice
- 1 tablespoon sour cream
- 2 avocados
- 1 tablespoon chopped fresh cilantro
- Salt to taste
- 1 tablespoon chives, minced

Directions:

1. Arrange Instant Pot over a dry platform in your kitchen. Open its top lid and switch it on.

2. In the pot, pour 1 cup water. Arrange a trivet or steamer basket inside that came with Instant Pot. Now place/arrange the egg over the trivet/basket.

3. Close top lid to create a locked chamber; make sure that safety valve is in locking position.

4. Find and press "MANUAL" cooking function; timer to 6 minutes with default "HIGH" pressure mode.

5. Allow the pressure to build to cook the ingredients.

6. After cooking time is over, press "CANCEL" setting. Find and press "QPR" cooking function. This setting is for quick release of inside pressure.

7. Cool down the eggs, peel and make halves.

8. Carefully remove yolks and add the yolks, and avocado into a bowl. With a fork, mash the mixture.

9. Mix in the remaining ingredients except for chives.

10. In a pastry bag, add the yolk mixture and pipe into egg white halves. Top with chives and serve.

Nutritional Values (Per Serving):

Calories – 232

Fat – 18g

Saturated Fat – 4g

Trans Fat – 0g

Carbohydrates – 6g

Fiber – 4g

Sodium – 183mg

Protein – 9g

Garlic Brussels Sprouts

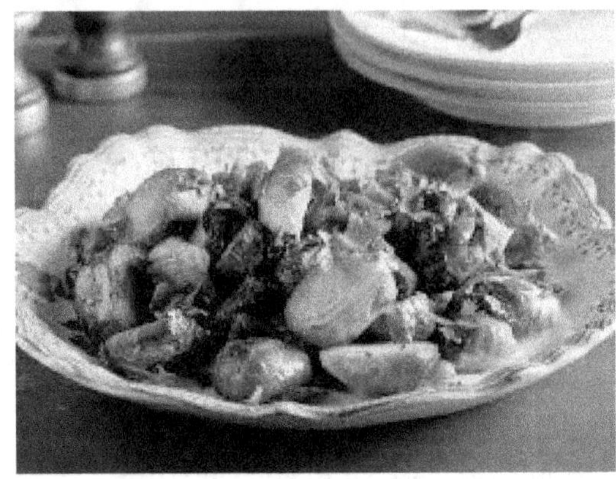

Prep Time: 8-10 min.

Cooking Time: 6 min.

Number of Servings: 3-4

Ingredients:

- 2 teaspoons minced garlic

- 1 pound Brussels sprout, trimmed and halved

- ½ cup water

- 2 tablespoons coconut oil

- ½ cup chopped yellow onion

- Salt and freshly (finely ground) black pepper, as per taste preference

Directions:

1. Arrange Instant Pot over a dry platform in your kitchen. Open its top lid and switch it on.

2. Find and press "SAUTE" cooking function; add the oil in it and allow it to heat.

3. In the pot, add the onions, garlic; cook (while stirring) until turns translucent and softened for around 2 minutes.

4. Add the ingredients; gently stir to mix well.

5. Close top lid to create a locked chamber; make sure that safety valve is in locking position.

6. Find and press "MANUAL" cooking function; timer to 2 minutes with default "HIGH" pressure mode.

7. Allow the pressure to build to cook the ingredients.

8. After cooking time is over, press "CANCEL" setting. Find and press "QPR" cooking function. This setting is for quick release of inside pressure.

9. Slowly open the lid, drain excess liquid; take out the cooked recipe in serving plates or serving bowls and enjoy the keto recipe.

Nutritional Values (Per Serving):

Calories - 128

Fat – 8g

Saturated Fat – 2g

Trans Fat – 0g

Carbohydrates – 7g

Fiber – 4g

Sodium – 163mg

Protein – 4g

Chapter 12: 7-day Keto Meal plan Recommendation

Day 1

Breakfast

Breakfast Mexican Omelet

Lunch

Mushroom Beef Chili

Afternoon

Parmesan Asparagus

Dinner

Turkey Tomato Meatballs

Day 2

Breakfast

Breakfast Casserole

Lunch

Chicken Spinach Curry

Afternoon

Spinach Mayo Dip

Dinner

Chicken Zucchini Pasta

Day 3

Breakfast

Cinnamon Chocolate Smoothie

Lunch

Super Herbed Fish

Afternoon

Garlic Brussels Sprouts

Dinner

Turkey Avocado Chili

Day 4

Breakfast

Black and Blue Smoothie

Lunch

Italian Eggplant Lasagna

Afternoon

Vanilla Cream Delight

Dinner

Chicken Relleno Casserole

Day 5

Breakfast

Cheese Blintz with Blueberries

Lunch

Cajun Rosemary Chicken

Afternoon

Tapioca Keto Pudding

Dinner

Cheesy Tomato Shrimp

Day 6

Breakfast

Almond Joy Microwave Muffin

Lunch

Chili Mac

Cauliflower Yogurt Mash Dip

Dinner

Chicken Chow Mein Stir Fry

Day 7

Breakfast

Butter Pecan Waffles

Lunch

Stuffed with Goat Cheese

Afternoon

Coconut Keto Pudding

Dinner

Salmon with Bok-Choy

Conclusion

There you have it – the ketogenic diet – easier with your assistant – the instant pot. At this point, you already know what it is, why it's good for you, how to implement or introduce the ketogenic diet, how to tell if you've already reached a state of ketosis. You also have sample meal plans, tips for staying ketogenic while eating out, and delicious recipes to try at home. You know enough about the ketogenic diet to start enjoying its benefits.

The ketogenic diet is a great way to watch pounds melt away, quickly and safely. Your own body turns into a fat burning machine, using up stores of fat rather than glucose from the food you're eating for energy.

At the same time, it protects your heart and other muscles from damage since you're feeding them nourishing, healthy oils and lots of needed protein.

For the ketogenic diet to work, you don't need to count calories and weigh or measure your food necessarily, but as with all eating plans, you need to be honest with yourself about what you're eating and how much.

I want you to remember though, no matter how much you try to lose that extra body fat, you must take your age into consideration. Especially if you have already passed middle age, you need to accept that you can no longer have the body you had when you were 20 or 30. Sometimes, in the quest to be our best, we may forget that we have a wholesome, working body – far more than a lot of people can say.

But don't lose heart, while the time to look your "best" may have passed, the time to just shed a few pounds, enjoy your body and live a healthier life is now! Try your best to find a balance between living healthily and being happy with the body you have. Make sure to follow this simple cookbook guide to help you lose weight and live an overall healthier lifestyle. So what are you waiting for – get slow cooking!

While virtually unlimited fats are allowed, it's good to get healthy, unsaturated fats that your body can easily digest and which won't clog your arteries; this means fats from fish, avocados, and peanuts, and olive oil. Lean protein choices are also better than fatty cuts of beef.

As with the rest of your food, you don't necessarily need to count carbohydrates, as long as you educate yourself about which foods are high in carbs and are sure to limit these in your diet.

If you do follow the ketogenic diet as recommended, you'll get a lean and toned physique in no time. You'll also calm your cravings, have a consistent source of energy, and won't feel fatigued throughout the day as you usually would.